CONTRACEPTION
TODAY
EIGHTH EDITION

CONTRACEPTION TODAY

EIGHTH EDITION

JOHN GUILLEBAUD

EMERITUS PROFESSOR OF FAMILY PLANNING AND REPRODUCTIVE HEALTH
UNIVERSITY COLLEGE LONDON, UK

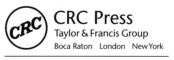

CRC Press
Taylor & Francis Group
Boca Raton London New York

CRC Press is an imprint of the
Taylor & Francis Group, an **informa** business

CRC Press
Taylor & Francis Group
6000 Broken Sound Parkway NW, Suite 300
Boca Raton, FL 33487-2742

© 2016 by Taylor & Francis Group, LLC
CRC Press is an imprint of Taylor & Francis Group, an Informa business

No claim to original U.S. Government works

Printed on acid-free paper
Version Date: 20151016

International Standard Book Number-13: 978-1-4987-1460-0 (Paperback)

Visit the Taylor & Francis Web site at
http://www.taylorandfrancis.com

and the CRC Press Web site at
http://www.crcpress.com

Contents

Preface

… how successful we have become. We as a species together with our cows, pigs etc, we are about 97 per cent of the biomass of all vertebrate species, meaning only 3 per cent are wild species.

Mathis Wackernagel, in *The Ecological Footprint,* **2005**

We have not inherited the earth from our grandparents, we have borrowed it from our grandchildren.

Kashmiri proverb

Family planning could bring more benefits to more people at less cost than any other single technology now available to the human race.

James Grant, UNICEF, 1992

Climate change absolutely must increase with growth in the numbers of climate changERS.

More Humanity with fewer Humans

Slogans of Population Matters/Optimum Population Trust

I have not seen an environmental problem that wouldn't be easier to solve with fewer people, or harder, and ultimately impossible, with ever more.

Sir David Attenborough, Patron of Population Matters

Born and reared in Burundi and Rwanda, countries whose recurrent agonies are in significant measure related to excessive population growth, I maintain that:

> Human needs along with those of all other species with which we share the Natural World will never be sustainably met on a finite planet without more concerned, non-coercive, action on human numbers.

No woman on earth who at time present wishes to exercise her human right to have the choice to control her fertility should be denied the means to do so, by barriers produced by any agency – whether through her partner's refusal, her society's pro-natalism, misinformation (sometimes deliberate), or lack of available, affordable and accessible contraceptive supplies and services. Family planning is preventive medicine *par excellence.*

Isn't overpopulation an overseas problem? Not so, in his or her lifetime, every new birth in the United Kingdom will, through the inevitable effluence of his or her affluence as a consumer, harm the environment – by climate change and in numerous other ways – as much as 30, or on some criteria 200, times more than births in Burundi or Bangladesh will ever do. We cannot be proud of our record in preventing teenage conceptions, and even in 2016 in all age groups conceptions still occur too often by chance rather than by choice. So we all have a part to play in ensuring that our grandchildren receive back their 'loan' in a halfway decent and long-term sustainable state. As a small but relevant contribution to that endeavour, I welcome this opportunity to bring a new edition of this pocketbook on contraception to general practitioners and nurses in primary care. (See also www.ecotimecapsule.com.)

I write, moreover, as one who is proud to have worked in general practice, as a locum in places as diverse as Barnsley, Cambridge, Luton and South London, and hence able to appreciate some of the satisfactions and the constraints of that role.

January 2016

Acknowledgements

I wish to thank numerous friends and colleagues in the United Kingdom and abroad working in relevant specialist and general practice – too many to mention all by name. Dr Diana Mansour and Professor Anne MacGregor deserve special mention, also Toni Belfield, formerly Head of Information at the UK Family Planning Association (FPA), and Robert Peden (of Taylor & Francis), who has guided this work through nearly all of its editions. I acknowledge repeated help from staff of the Clinical Effectiveness Unit of the Faculty of Sexual and Reproductive Health (FSRH) and, over many years, from senior medical and nursing staff at the Margaret Pyke Centre (MPC), London, and in Oxford within the Family Planning Service and at the Elliot-Smith Vasectomy Clinic. Finally, I am also grateful to some of our clients for the insights they have given me over the years.

DISCLAIMER

Use of several brand names throughout this book does not *per se* imply any endorsement, they are only used for ease of reference.

Introduction

General practitioners (GPs) and practice nurses are often best placed to offer good contraceptive advice because they already know the patient's health and family circumstances. Some practices are excellent; others provide little beyond oral contraception and devote insufficient time and skill to counselling. The 2002 Sexual Health Strategy established that primary care should always supply at least 'Level 1' basic contraceptive services and should also consider supplying services at 'Level 2'. These include all the long-acting reversible contraceptive methods (LARCs). The National Institute for Health and Care Excellence (NICE) clinical guideline (www.nice.org.uk/guidance/cg30) draws attention to the many contraceptive (and sometimes non-contraceptive) advantages of these methods, comprising injectables, implants, the latest copper-banded intrauterine devices (IUDs) and the levonorgestrel intrauterine systems (LNG-IUSs). If LARCs are not supplied on site, practices should have referral arrangements in place for the LARCs, agreed to be within 24 hours for copper IUDs as emergency contraception (EC); and also when appropriate for Level 3 services such as male and female sterilization and medical or surgical abortion.

Iatrogenic ('doctor-caused') pregnancies are a reality. They result from avoidable errors or omissions on the part of service providers, especially the omission of sufficient time for the consultation.

Women choosing their first-ever 'medical' contraceptive need more than the usual 10 minutes available in most surgeries. 'The minimum recommended consultation time for a routine new appointment is 20 minutes and the minimum recommended time for a routine follow-up appointment is 10 minutes'. This time can be shared between a clinical team e.g. nurse plus doctor (www.fsrh.org/pdfs/ServiceStandardsWorkload.pdf).

Writing as 'an ex-GP', 20 minutes is obviously daunting yet not unreasonable, when one considers the ground to be covered, say for a first-time Pill user (see p. 55). An arrangement that works well in some practices is to offer routinely a second 10- to 15-minute consultation within the same week, either at the end of a surgery or with the practice nurse.

Much of this work can – indeed, should – be the responsibility of practice nurses trained in family planning, usually with a gain rather than a loss in standards. Practice is changing fast, with more use of patient group directions and more nurse practitioners who are prescribers. Some changes since the last edition are that nurses, like doctors, can train with the Faculty of Sexual and Reproductive Healthcare (FSRH) and obtain the NDFSRH, not essentially different from the doctors' DFSRH, and can also acquire the LOCs (letters of competence), for intrauterine and subdermal contraceptives (full details at www.fsrh.org/pages/Diploma_of_the_FSRH.asp). Even without this certification, any good 'mainstream' practice nurse may perform the following delegated functions appropriately and well:

- Taking sexual and medical histories, discussing choices (using UK Family Planning Association leaflets).
- Pill teaching.
- Pill issuing/reissuing and emergency Pill issuing – given fully agreed and audited patient group directions.
- Pill monitoring, including migraine assessment and blood pressure (BP).
- Giving contraceptive injections: depot medroxyprogesterone acetate (DMPA; Depo-Provera® or Sayana® Press).
- IUD and IUS checking, including eliciting cervical excitation tenderness at vaginal examination.
- Cervical smear taking.

All GPs and practice nurses working in reproductive health need to be comfortable when faced by the often complex psychosexual and emotional factors involved in the use of contraception. Clinicians should be sensitive to hidden signals in this area. Relevant training courses are run by the Institute of Psychosexual Medicine (www.ipm.org.uk), the College for Sexual and Relationship Therapy (www.cosrt.org.uk) and Relate (www.relate.org.uk).

Doctors or nurses should back their counselling with good literature. Although some manufacturers have improved their patient information leaflets (PILs), the latest FPA leaflets are user friendly, accurate and comprehensive. The one called 'Your Contraceptive Choices' tabulates all the important methods, both reversible and permanent, and can help when read in the waiting room before counselling. The leaflets on individual methods can best be downloaded as pdfs by new users from the FPA website in up-to-date versions. Together with accurate contemporary records, leaflets – added to, as is sometimes needed, if an intended use is evidence based but not yet licensed (p. 165) – provide strong medico-legal backup for practitioners who may be asked to justify their actions in the event of litigation. PILs are an essential supplement to – but by no means a replacement for – time spent with the healthcare practitioner.

CHOICE OF METHOD

Most women who seek contraception are healthy and young, and they present fewer problems than those who are more than 35 years old, teenagers and those with intercurrent disease. There is a tendency for sterilization procedures to be demanded at too early an age. This is partly because the Pill is too often seen as synonymous with contraception, and we as providers have not been informing women about the many new or improved reversible alternatives, about which there is still much mythology and ignorance. In Figure 1, the methods at bottom left are known collectively as the LARCs – the

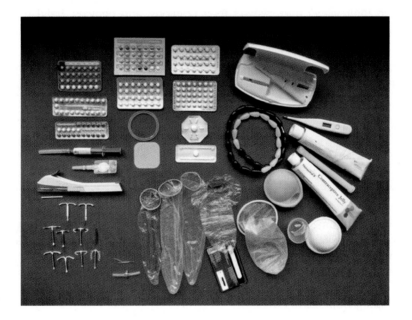

Figure 1

The choice of methods in the United Kingdom (2015). (Courtesy of Professor Anne MacGregor, and Colin Parker of Durbin PLC.) The products shown are as follows, in a clockwise spiral, starting from the bottom left-hand corner: various copper intrauterine devices (labelled at p. 107), and above them a 52-mg and a 13.5-mg levonorgestrel intrauterine system. Above that is a Nexplanon® and its inserter, then the injectable depot medroxyprogesterone acetate in two forms, Sayana® Press (subcutaneous) (p. 85) and Depo-Provera® (intramuscular). Above that are combined oral contraceptives Logynon®, Millinette 20/75® and (top left) Microgynon® ED. Continuing clockwise are Qlaira® (p. 64) above Zoely® (p. 64), and then the desogestrel progestogen-only Pill above Norgeston®. Top right is Persona® (p. 155), and a fertility thermometer. Below them are CycleBeads® (p. 154) and tubes of spermicide, Caya® gel and Gygel® with an applicator (p. 152). The Caya diaphragm® is just above a FemCap® with (bottom right) a standard diaphragm. Continuing clockwise is first a Femidom® (p. 150) and then assorted plastic then latex condoms (p. 149). Then comes a Filshie® female sterilization clip with, above it, an Essure® tubal insert (p. 157). Above the latex condoms, the spiral finishes centrally with an Evra® Patch under a NuvaRing® (pp. 68–71) and the emergency contraception methods ellaOne® above Levonelle 1500® (p. 135).

LNG-IUS, the banded copper IUDs, injectables and the latest implants. All of these can be seen as 'in the same ballpark' as reversible female sterilization.

THE YOUNG

I am opposed to 'sex education'! This is because I support – as we all should – sex and *relationships* education (SRE). When seeking advice on sex, relationships, contraception, pregnancy and parenthood, young people are entitled to accessible, confidential, non-judgemental and unbiased support and guidance, recognizing the diversity of their cultural and faith traditions. We should listen to their views and respect their opinions and choices. Valid choices include waiting ('saving sex'), as well as having (safer and contracepted) sex.

It is not a good idea to have sex only because:
- someone else wants you to.
- someone says he or she will leave you if you don't.
- all your friends say they are doing it.
- you feel too scared to say 'no'.
- OR: when it just doesn't seem right to you (with this person or now).

From www.likeitis.org, slightly altered.

However, because they may often 'get away with it' in one or more cycles, all too often the young do not seek advice until they have already conceived. Preventing this depends on the best use of available contraceptive technology, as in the box in this section on methods for teenagers, but also on *much more than that*. See the excellent guidance at www.fsrh.org/pdfs/ceuGuidanceYoungPeople2010.pdf.

Education for both genders must promote the societal norm that, unless conception is planned, sex may be a feature of a good relationship only when and if adequate contraception exists. In the Netherlands this norm, backed by peer pressure from teens themselves, leads to far fewer teenage conceptions than in the United Kingdom, despite some improvement here since 2000.

In this age group, easier access to EC is an obvious priority. We also await improvements in the fully 'forgettable' methods where (in contrast to the Pill) non-pregnancy is the default state. We already do have the LARCs; injectables and implants (often best used in this order; see p. 101) are usually preferable to copper IUDs, although these are only relatively contraindicated (p. 129); and that option should surely be offered as EC more often than it is (p. 137). One of the LNG-IUSs may also be appropriate for some young people, although not post-coitally (p. 127). See the box (p. 5) on methods for teenagers.

List of methods for teenagers in order of preference

As always, the user is the chooser: the provider should move down the list until the user reaches her choice.

1. DMPA – intramuscular or subcutaneous according to choice – with plan to move on to Nexplanon when amenorrhoeic (p. 101) or later, when she agrees.
2. Nexplanon or Jaydess® IUS, but unless seen in first week of a cycle and with facilities to fit at once, quick-starting first a progestin-only pill (POP) or combined oral contraceptive (COC) and proceeding to fit approximately 3 weeks later at everyone's convenience (see 'ploy' on p. 161) after a pregnancy test as indicated.
3. Copper IUD, commonly because she needed EC and ideally using the T-Safe Cu 380A®, often in its Mini TT 380 Slimline® version (see p. 137).
4. Desogestrel POP or 20 μg COC usually Loestrin 20®, taken as the tailored pill, continuously (p. 49). (These are acceptable for teens because both have no contraception-weakening pill-free intervals (PFIs); see p. 43.)
5. Microgynon, in its ED form with 7 placebos for the PFI (tip: offer 'Sunday start', as at Table 7 [pp. 56–7], if acceptable).
6. NuvaRing®, pricey but good because it approaches the 'forgetability' of being a LARC.

Notes:

If hormonal EC required at first visit, quick-starting of the new method would often be wise (no. 3 is already a quick-start method, of course), though special terms apply if UPA EC is selected (pp. 141–2).

Plus, outside of monogamy, supply or advise condoms as well, and ensure availability of all three EC options.

When counselling teens (or others) who are requesting surgical termination of pregnancy, discuss in advance the logical option of IUD or IUS insertion at the time (as at p. 131);

Observe the priority in this list that is given to the LARCs; and the low status of COCs (and then best given continuously or at least as ED versions!).

COC, combined oral contraceptive; DMPA, depot medroxyprogesterone acetate; EC, emergency contraception; IUD, intrauterine device; IUS, intrauterine system; LARC, long-acting reversible contraceptive method; PFI, pill-free interval; POP, progestogen-only pill.

In patients less than 16 years of age, it is entirely appropriate – so long as it is done opportunely, non-judgementally and never patronizingly – to present the emotional as well as medical advantages of delaying coitarche ('saving sex') and then of mutually faithful relationships. However, even if that is medically the 'best', when rejected it must not become the enemy of the 'good', a category that surely includes contraception combined with age-appropriate SRE – the latter ideally being started at home by the parent(s) and not just left to schools. Legally, following the guidance presented here, in the decision to prescribe a medical method of contraception, an attempt should first be made to seek parental support. However, if the young person

Confidentiality and related issues
- Is your practice SRH service's confidentiality policy explicit, and implicit (i.e. does it feel cast-iron to her/him)?
- Does the young person (<16 or not) understand her/his rights – 'including the right not to have or delay having sex … and how to negotiate safer sex'?
- Might there be abuse or coercion? School exclusion and involvement of social services are useful markers of this. Check the girl's partner's age – and hers (is she truly *not* younger than 13?).
- If it therefore becomes necessary for others or other agencies to become involved, always inform the young person.
- All SRH services 'should have a named person identified as the local lead for child protection'.
- 'First intercourse is often associated with regret, feeling pressured and alcohol consumption.'
From www.fsrh.org/pdfs/ceuGuidanceYoungPeople2010.pdf.

refuses to allow this, it is indubitably good practice to initiate a suitable 'medical' contraceptive, ideally an LARC.

There is a useful mnemonic for the 'Fraser guidelines' regarding those less than 16 years old. These guidelines still have relevance, although they were issued back in 1985, shortly after the Gillick case.

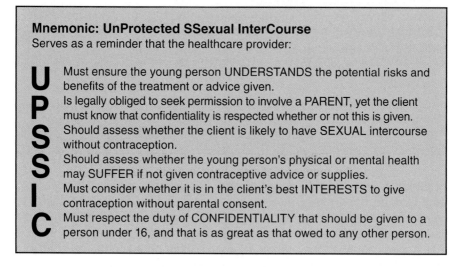

Mnemonic: UnProtected SSexual InterCourse
Serves as a reminder that the healthcare provider:

U Must ensure the young person UNDERSTANDS the potential risks and benefits of the treatment or advice given.

P Is legally obliged to seek permission to involve a PARENT, yet the client must know that confidentiality is respected whether or not this is given.

S Should assess whether the client is likely to have SEXUAL intercourse without contraception.

S Should assess whether the young person's physical or mental health may SUFFER if not given contraceptive advice or supplies.

I Must consider whether it is in the client's best INTERESTS to give contraception without parental consent.

C Must respect the duty of CONFIDENTIALITY that should be given to a person under 16, and that is as great as that owed to any other person.

If the foregoing guidance is followed, in utmost good faith, the prescription of a medical method of contraception will never be seen as aiding or abetting the commission of what persists in law as the crime of underage sex.

SEXUALLY TRANSMITTED INFECTIONS

Taking a quick but matter-of-fact sexual history need not be stressful. It should be seen as part of the consultation for all contraceptives, not just the intrauterine ones.

In context (of discussion about sex and contraception), ask:

- 'When did you last have sex?' and then immediately
- 'When did you last have sex with anybody different?'

Much can be learnt at once from this pair of open questions, whether the response is 'about 21 years ago' or say '3 months ago'. If the latter, it now becomes unthreatening (unlike other approaches) to go on and clarify whether this was a change of partner or 'a one night stand' – and whether there have been others in the past year. Getting a handle on whether the woman's partner himself is monogamous or otherwise can be tricky, but if tactfully asked, she may, sometimes, have a pretty good idea.

In the United Kingdom, higher risk of infection, particularly with *Chlamydia trachomatis,* applies to women less than 25 years old and/or presenting with the request for EC. However, a good history taken as described earlier, suggests an even greater likelihood of a positive result if there has been:

- a partner change in the previous 12 weeks.
- more than one partner in the past 12 months.
- any history of having tests at a sexual health clinic.

Advise all patients about minimizing their risk of sexually transmitted infections (STIs), including human immunodeficiency virus (HIV). If when counselling an individual the 'selling' of monogamy fails, it is essential to promote the condom as an addition to the selected contraceptive, whenever (now or later) there may be an infection risk – the so-called double-Dutch approach.

Features of the ideal contraceptive
- 100 per cent effective (with the default state as contraception).
- 100 per cent convenient (can forget about it, not coitally related).
- 100 per cent safe, free of adverse side effects (neither risk nor nuisance).
- 100 per cent reversible, ideally by self.
- 100 per cent maintenance free, meaning it needs absolutely no medical or provider intervention (with potential pain or discomfort), whether initially or ongoing or to achieve reversal.
- 100 per cent protective against sexually transmitted infections.
- Having other non-contraceptive benefits, especially to reduce the dis-'eases' of the menstrual cycle.
- Inexpensive, easy to distribute.
- Acceptable to every culture, religion and political view.
- Used by or at least obviously visible to the woman, who most needs to know it has worked!

No available method meets all the criteria in the foregoing box, although the LNG-IUS is closest.

RELATIVE EFFECTIVENESS OF THE AVAILABLE METHODS

Failure rates of methods are usually expressed as per 100 woman-years. A figure of 10 per 100 woman-years for a 'perfect user' (see later) means that in a population of 100 users, 10 women might be expected to conceive in the first year of use of the method; or, notionally, 1 woman would have an 'evens' chance of having an unplanned pregnancy after 10 years of its use. In Table 1, 'Perfect use' means the method is used both consistently and correctly, whereas 'Typical use' means what it says and is obviously hugely dependent on characteristics (e.g. age, social class, acceptability of conception) of the population studied. Note the great difference in percentage conceiving after 1 year between the two types of use for the combined Pill (0.3 vs. 9). The data in this table are from the United States, but the 'Perfect use' data are usable for comparing methods in any setting.

Continuation rates also vary even among 'perfect' users and in general are much higher for the LARCs.

Table 1

Percentage of women experiencing an unintended pregnancy during the first year of use of contraception

Method	Percentage of women with an unintended pregnancy within the first year of use		Percentage of women continuing use at 1 year
	Typical use[a]	Perfect use[b]	Continuation rate[c]
No method	85	85	
Spermicides[d]	28	18	42
Withdrawal	22	4	46
Fertility awareness–based methods[e]	24		47
Standard days method		5	
Ovulation method		3	
Sponge			
Parous women	24	20	36
Nulliparous women	12	9	
Diaphragm plus spermicide	12	6	57
Condom			
Female	21	5	41
Male	18	2	43
Combined Pill and POP	9	0.3	67
Evra patch and NuvaRing	9	0.3	
Depo-Provera	6	0.2	56
Intrauterine device			
T-Safe Cu 380[f]	0.8	0.6	78
Mirena® (LNG-IUS20)	0.2	0.2	80
Nexplanon	0.05	0.05	84
Female sterilization	0.5	0.5	100
Male sterilization	0.15	0.10	100

Data from United States: Trussell J. *Contraception* 2011;83:397–404. www.ncbi.nlm.nih.gov/pmc/articles/PMC3638209/table/T1 (available, open access, to review the assumptions made).

For couples who initiate use of a method (not necessarily for the first time), in each of columns 2 and 3, the percentage is shown of those who experience an accidental pregnancy during the first year if they do not stop use for any other reason.

[a]Column 2 shows these rates for *typical* users.

[b]Column 3 gives the failure rates for couples who use each method *perfectly* (both consistently and correctly).

[c]Column 4 shows, among couples attempting to avoid pregnancy, the percentage who continue to use a method for 1 year.

[d]Foams, creams, gels, vaginal suppositories and vaginal film (Gygel available in the United Kingdom).

[e]The Ovulation method is based on evaluation of cervical mucus. The Standard Days method avoids intercourse on cycle days 8 through 19 (p. 154).

[f]Marketed as ParaGard® in United States.

ELIGIBILITY CRITERIA FOR CONTRACEPTIVES

The WHO system for classifying contraindications

This excellent scheme (first devised in a small WHO workshop that I attended in 1994, in Atlanta) is more fully described in the document issued by WHO, *Medical Eligibility Criteria for Contraceptive Use,* fifth edition (Geneva: WHO, 2015), which is referred to from now on as WHOMEC. This is dark blue, and its companion volume (green) is *Selected Practice Recommendations for Contraceptive Use* (Geneva: WHO, 2004), generally referred to as WHOSPR. They are readily downloadable from www.who.int/reproductivehealth/topics/family_planning/en/index.html (click on the relevant icons for either volume). Both of these documents are evidence based, where evidence exists.

The FSRH's Clinical Effectiveness Unit has since developed a UK version (UKMEC) of WHOMEC, which adjusts for UK practice and so differs slightly – therefore in most (but not quite all) cases being more closely congruent with this book. UKMEC is available on the FSRH website www.fsrh.org/pdfs/UKMEC2009.pdf.

WHOMEC and UKMEC classify eligibility for contraceptive methods into four categories, as shown in the following box:

WHO classification of contraindications
The A to D designation is the author's parallel aide-memoire for the significance of each category:
1. A condition for which there is no restriction for the use of the contraceptive method.
   'A' is for **Always Usable**.
2. A condition where the advantages of the method generally outweigh the theoretical or proven risks.
   'B' is for **Broadly Usable, Be alert** (for any future added risk).

   ****

3. A condition where the theoretical or proven risks usually outweigh the advantages, so an alternative method is usually preferred. Yet, respecting the patient or client's autonomy, if she accepts the risks and rejects or should not use relevant alternatives, given the risks of pregnancy, the method can be used with caution or sometimes with additional monitoring. In sum, 'C' is for **Caution/Counselling**, if used at all.
4. A condition that represents an unacceptable health risk.
   'D' is for **DO NOT USE**, at all.

The most useful feature of the classification is the separation into two categories of 'relative' contraindication (WHO 2 and 3), with the 'strong relative' ones (WHO 3) *below the line*, thus implying that they normally indicate non-use of the method.

Clinical judgement is required, always in consultation with the contraceptive user, especially (1) in all WHO 3 conditions or (2) if more than one condition applies. As a working rule, two WHO 2 conditions usually move the situation to WHO 3; and if any WHO 3 condition applies, the addition of either a 2 or a 3 condition normally means WHO 4 (i.e. 'Do not use').

For all the medical methods described in the rest of this book, the listed absolute or relative contraindications are based on the foregoing scheme. Prescribers often have to make a decision (in consultation with the woman or couple) despite a frustrating absence of good evidence.

What follows is the best interim guidance, pending more data, according to this author's judgement after assessing the evidence and the views of WHOMEC and UKMEC, if available. Note that these bodies have yet to give their verdict on some issues.

To avoid confusion, here, WHO 1 to 4 is used by me as the scale, according to the WHO's categorization schema, with the chosen category most often but not always identical to that currently advised in this country by UKMEC. A number (i.e. 1 to 4) preceded by UKMEC signifies the category actually selected by the UK committee concerned. The few usually small differences in this text from UKMEC and/or WHO are identified by (JG), or 'in my view'.

Final introductory points are as follows:

1. The manufacturers' Summary of Product Characteristics (SPCs) and PILs may also differ (from WHOMEC, from UKMEC and from what is said here).
2. Use of some brand names here does not imply their endorsement; they are used only for ease of reference.
3. There is a Glossary in the Appendix for all abbreviations.

CHC is not a typo for COC (combined oral contraceptive(s)); it means combined hormonal contraceptive(s), the subject of the next chapter, and includes along with oral Pills, contraceptive patches and rings (Evra and NuvaRing). Although the evidence base is far stronger for COCs, the majority of the statements about them will also apply to the other CHCs. Indeed, when reading the next chapter practically every statement about 'the COC' or 'the Pill' can be assumed to apply to patches and rings (i.e. to all CHCs), except in obvious circumstances relating to the different routes of administration.

Combined hormonal contraception

The invaluable Guidance document of the Faculty of Sexual and Reproductive Health, available from the FSRH at www.fsrh.org/pdfs/CEU GuidanceCombinedHormonalContraception.pdf, is highly recommended, to amplify this chapter's content, with references. Note *combined hormonal contraception* in the URL which, like this chapter, relates generally to CHCs and not just COCs.

COMBINED ORAL CONTRACEPTIVES

Mechanism of action

The COC Pills currently available in the United Kingdom are shown in Table 2. They combine an estrogen (ethinylestradiol [EE] in all cases but three) with one of nine progestogens.

Aside from secondary contraceptive effects on the cervical mucus and to impede implantation, COCs primarily prevent ovulation. This makes the method highly effective in 'perfect' use (see Table 1), but it removes the normal menstrual cycle and replaces it with a cycle that is user produced and based only on the end organ (i.e. the endometrium). So the withdrawal bleeding has minimal medical significance and can be deliberately postponed or made infrequent or never occurring at week-ends (see Footnote b of Figure 7, p. 57), or abolished (e.g. tricycling and 365/365 Pill-taking – discussed later); and if it fails to occur, once pregnancy is excluded, this poses no problem. The Pill-free time is the contraception-deficient time, which has great relevance to advice for the maintenance of COC efficacy (see later).

Benefits versus risks

Capable of providing virtually 100 per cent protection from unwanted pregnancy and taken at a time unconnected with sexual activity, the COC provides enormous reassurance by the associated regular, short, light and usually painless withdrawal bleeding at the end of the 21-day pack. Inevitably, most of this section will focus on possible risks and hazards associated with taking the

Table 2
Formulations of UK combined oral contraceptives (24/7 regimens unless otherwise stated)

Pill type	Brand names available (in United Kingdom[a])	Estrogen (µg)	Progestogen (µg)
Monophasic			
Ethinylestradiol/ Norethisterone	Loestrin® 20	20	1000 Norethisterone acetate
	Loestrin® 30	30	1500 Norethisterone acetate[b]
	Brevinor®	35	500 Norethisterone
	Ovysmen®		
	Norimin®	35	1000 Norethisterone
Ethinylestradiol/ levonorgestrel	Microgynon® 30 (and ED version) Rigevidon® Levest® Ovranette® others	30	150
Ethinylestradiol/ desogestrel	Mercilon® Gedarel® 20/150	20	150
	Marvelon® Gedarel® 30/150	30	150
Ethinylestradiol/ gestodene	Femodette® 20/75 Sunya® 20/75 Millinette® 20/75	20	75
	Femodene® (and ED version) Katya® 30/75 Millinette® 30/75	30	75
Ethinylestradiol/ norgestimate	Cilest®	35	250
Ethinylestradiol/ drospirenone	Daylette® [24/4ED]	20	3000
	Yasmin®	30	3000
Ethinylestradiol/ cyproterone acetate (co-cyprindiol)	Dianette® Clairette® Acnocin® Cicafem®	35	2000
Mestranol[c]/ norethisterone	Norinyl-1®	50	1000
Bi/triphasic			
Ethinylestradiol/ norethisterone	BiNovum®	35 35	500⎫833[d] (7 tabs) 1000⎭ (14 tabs)
	Synphase®	35 35 35	500⎫ (7 tabs) 1000⎬714[d] (9 tabs) 500⎭ (5 tabs)
	TriNovum®	35 35 35	500⎫ (7 tabs) 750⎬750[d] (7 tabs) 1000⎭ (7 tabs)
Ethinylestradiol/ levonorgestrel	Logynon® (and ED) TriRegol®	30⎫ 40⎬32[d] 30⎭	50⎫ (6 tabs) 75⎬92[d] (5 tabs) 125⎭ (10 tabs)

(Continued)

Table 2 (Continued)
Formulations of UK combined oral contraceptives (24/7 regimens unless otherwise stated)

Pill type	Brand names available (in United Kingdom[a])	Estrogen (μg)	Progestogen (μg)	
Ethinylestradiol/ gestodene	Triadene®	30 ⎤ 40 ⎬ 32[d] 30 ⎦	50 ⎤ 70 ⎬ 79[d] 100 ⎦	(6 tabs) (5 tabs) (10 tabs)
Estradiol valerate/ dienogest (*with natural estrogen*)	Qlaira®	3000 2000 2000 1000 Inert	Nil 2000 3000 Nil Inert	(2 tabs) (5 tabs) (17 tabs) (2 tabs) (2 tabs)
Estradiol hemihydrate/ nomegestrol acetate (*with natural estrogen, monophasic, 4-day PFI*)	Zoely® [24/4ED]	1500	2000	

[a]Other names in use worldwide are on the website www.ippf.org.
[b]Converted to norethisterone as the active metabolite.
[c]Has to be converted to ethinylestradiol, approximately 35 μg, as active estrogen, so Norinyl-1 approximates to Norimin (see text).
[d]Equivalent daily doses per formulation in these columns, for comparison with monophasic brands.

Pill, but the positive aspects should not be forgotten; they are listed in the box that follows. Although some of these findings await full confirmation, the good news is rarely mentioned while the suspected risks are widely publicized and often overdramatized.

Space does not allow full discussion of all the work that has been published in the half-century during which the Pill has been available in this country. Practitioners should form their own opinions of the risks and benefits by their own readings, but the following may help to summarize present medical opinion on which contemporary prescription of the Pill is based.

The data presented here have been derived from the prospective Royal College of General Practitioners (RCGP), Oxford/Family Planning Association (FPA) and US Nurses Studies, supplemented by numerous case-control studies and a few randomized controlled trials (RCTs) conducted by WHO and other bodies.

Contraceptive benefits of COCs
- Effectiveness.
- Convenience, not intercourse related.
- Reversibility.

Non-contraceptive benefits of COCs

These benefits at times may provide the principal indications for use of the method (e.g. in the treatment of severe primary dysmenorrhoea in a not-yet sexually active teenager).

- Reduction of most menstrual cycle disorders: less heavy bleeding, therefore less anaemia and less dysmenorrhoea; regular bleeding, the timing of which can be controlled (no Pill taker ever needs to have Pill 'periods' at weekends); fewer symptoms of premenstrual tension overall; no ovulation pain.
- Reduced risk of cancer of the ovary, cancer of the endometrium and also, according to latest data, colorectal cancer.
- Fewer functional ovarian cysts because associated abnormal ovulation is prevented.
- Fewer extrauterine pregnancies because normal ovulation is inhibited.
- Reduction in pelvic inflammatory disease (PID).
- Reduction in benign breast disease (BBD).
- Fewer symptomatic fibroids.
- Probable reduction in thyroid disease, whether overactivity or underactivity.
- Probable reduction in risk of rheumatoid arthritis.
- Fewer sebaceous disorders, especially acne (with estrogen-dominant COCs such as Marvelon and Yasmin).
- Possible reduced risk of endometriosis (a potential benefit probably not as well realized as it would be if the Pill were more commonly taken in a bleeding-free regimen).
- Continuous use certainly beneficial in long-term suppression of established endometriosis.
- Possibly fewer duodenal ulcers (not well established).
- Reduction in *Trichomonas vaginalis* infections.
- Possible lower incidence of toxic shock syndrome.
- No toxicity in overdose.
- Some obvious beneficial social effects, to balance the suggested negative social effects.

Even as we turn to unwanted effects, it is reassuring that, based, among other things, on the regular reports of the RCGP study ever since it began in 1968, COCs have their main (small) effect on every known associated cause of mortality during current use and for some (variable) time thereafter. The excess thrombotic risk has probably vanished by 4 weeks, and by 10 years after use ceases, all-cause mortality in past users is lower than or (allowing for healthy-user bias) certainly indistinguishable from that in never users.

Tumour risk

No medication continues to receive so much scrutiny and investigation as the Pill. Fears have been expressed for many years about its possible connection with breast, cervical and (rare) primary liver cancers.

Breast cancer

The incidence of this disease is high, and therefore it must inevitably be expected to develop in women whether they take COCs or not. Given that the recognized risk factors include early menarche and late age of first birth, use by young women was rightly bound to receive scientific scrutiny. The literature to date has been copious, complex, confusing and often contradictory!

The 1996 publication by the Collaborative Group on Hormonal Factors in Breast Cancer reanalysed original data relating to more than 3000 women with breast cancer and more than 100 000 controls from 54 studies in 25 countries. This represents epidemiological data from 90 per cent of the world. The reanalysis showed disappearance of the risk in ex-users, but recency of use of the COC was shown to be the most important factor, with the odds ratio (OR) unaffected by age of initiation or discontinuation, use before or after first full-term pregnancy, duration of use, or dose. The main findings are summarized in Table 3. Figure 2 shows that the background risk of cancer in women younger than 35 years is, fortunately, very small. Hence, for the age group of women who most often use the method, the absolute numbers affected even for current users with the highest added risk in Table 3 are actually small.

Table 3
The increased risk of developing breast cancer while taking the Pill and in the 10 years after stopping

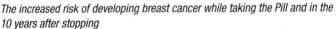

User status	Percentage increased risk
Current user	24%
1–4 years after stopping	16%
5–9 years after stopping	7%
10 plus years an ex-user	No significant excess risk

Source: From Collaborative Group on Hormonal Factors in Breast Cancer. *Lancet* 1996;347:1713–1727.

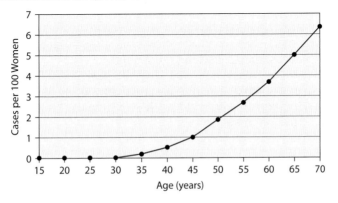

Figure 2
Background risk: cumulative number of breast cancers per 100 women, by age. (From statement by the Faculty of Family Planning—now FSRH—June 1996.)

A 2002 study of 4575 patients with breast cancer and matched cancer-free controls in the United States was congruent with this finding and particularly reassuring in that there was nothing to suggest the so-called time-bomb problem: namely, despite 75 per cent exposure to the COC in the population, there was no persistence of risk in long-time ex-users when they reached ages with much higher incidence of this cancer, as shown in Figure 2. This finding remains valid to date (2015), after taking account of all subsequent reports.

COC-users can be reassured that:
- Although the small increase in breast cancer risk for women on the Pill noted in previous studies is confirmed, the OR of 1.24 signifies an increase of 24 per cent only while women are taking the COC; this percentage diminishes to zero after COC discontinuation, over the next few years.
- Beyond 10 years after stopping, there is no detectable increase in breast cancer risk for former Pill users.
- The cancers diagnosed in women who use or have ever used COCs are clinically less advanced than those in women who have never used the Pill, and these tumours are less likely to have spread beyond the breast.
- These risks are not associated with duration of use, or the dose or type of hormone in the COC, and there is no synergism with other risk factors for breast cancer (e.g. family history).
- If 1000 women use the Pill till age 35 years, then by age 45 this model (which itself is a 'worst-case scenario') shows there will be, in all, 11 cases of breast cancer. Importantly, however, as displayed in Figure 3, only one of these cases is extra (i.e. Pill related), the others would have arisen anyway, in a control group of 1000 never users.

Clinical implications

Discussion of this issue should be initiated opportunely – not necessarily at the first visit if not raised by the woman – along with encouragement to report promptly any unusual changes in their breasts at any time in the future ('breast awareness'). The balancing protective effects against other malignancies (see later) should always be mentioned.

The known contraceptive and non-contraceptive benefits of COCs may seem so great to many (but not to all) as to compensate for almost any likely lifetime excess risk of breast cancer.

- What about Pill use by older women? There is no change in relative risk, but an increased attributable risk (3 extra cases per 1000 for 10th year ex-users stopping at 45 years and now 55 years old, instead of the foregoing 1 extra case per 1000 for 10th year ex-users now 45 years old). This needs explaining and may be acceptable to many, given the balancing (see later) from the well-established protection against cancers of the ovary, endometrium, colon and rectum – and their incidence also increases with age. However, the majority of women would now probably prefer one of the newer options available (such as the IUS or banded copper IUD; see later).

- Women with benign breast disease (BBD) or with a family history of a young first-degree relative with breast cancer before age 40 years have a larger background risk than the generality of women – but only the same as women slightly older than their current age who are free of the risk factor. This equates to a small shift of the curve to the left in Figure 2. Hence UKMEC classifies both these conditions as WHO 1 for the COC (no restriction on use).
- If the woman with BBD had a breast biopsy, the histology report should be obtained: if the rare pre-malignant epithelial atypia was found, the COC should not be used (WHO 4).
- Carriers of known gene mutations (e.g. *BRCA1*) associated with this cancer should also normally avoid the COC (WHO 3).
- If a woman develops carcinoma of the breast, COCs should be discontinued, and women with a personal history of this cancer should avoid COCs (WHO 4). COC use after 5 years of remission is UKMEC 3.

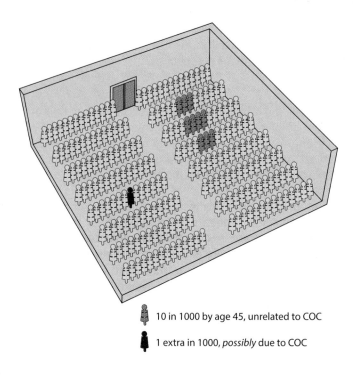

👤 10 in 1000 by age 45, unrelated to COC

👤 1 extra in 1000, *possibly* due to COC

Figure 3
Cumulative incidence of breast cancer during and after use of COC until age 35 years.

Cervical cancer

Human papillomavirus (HPV), especially types 16 and 18, appears to be the principal carcinogen for this cancer, which is clearly transmitted sexually. Systematic reviews of studies led to the conclusion that the COC acts as a cofactor, possibly speeding transition through the stages of cervical intraepithelial neoplasia (CIN). The raised OR is further increased with increasing durations of use. As a cofactor, the COC acts similarly to, but is certainly weaker than, cigarette smoking.

Clinical implications
- Prescribers must ensure that COC users and ex-users are adequately screened following agreed guidelines. Even if they also smoke, a 3-yearly cervical smear frequency starting from age 25 years, as in national guidelines, is still believed to suffice to identify – and then treat appropriately – most (although no screening programme can have 100 per cent success) lesions in the pre-invasive stages, before actual cancer develops.
- It is acceptable practice (WHO 2) to continue COC use during the careful monitoring of any abnormality, or after definitive treatment of CIN.

The relative importance of any adverse effect of the COC on cervical cancer should be further minimized in future by widespread HPV vaccination to reduce the incidence, as well as HPV triage for borderline and mild dyskaryosis to improve pre-cancer detection.

Liver tumours

COC use increases the relative risk of benign adenoma or hamartoma, either of which can cause pain or rarely a haemoperitoneum. Most reported cases have been in long-term users of relatively high-dose Pills that are now not used. Moreover, the background incidence is so small (1 to 3 per 1 million women per year) that the COC-attributable risk is minimal.

Case-control studies support the view that the rare primary hepatocellular carcinoma is also minimally less rare in COC users than in controls. Yet there is reassuring contrary evidence to the association being causative, namely that, although this cancer is usually rapidly fatal, the death rate from it has not changed detectably in either the United States or Sweden, where the COC has been widely used since the 1960s. Moreover, there is no evidence of synergism with either cirrhosis or hepatitis B liver infection.

Clinical implications
A past history of liver tumour (benign or malignant) is WHO 4 for any CHC but WHO 3 for other forms of hormonal contraception.

Choriocarcinoma or other forms of gestational trophoblastic disease – no problem

In the presence of active trophoblastic disease, early studies from the United Kingdom showed that chemotherapy for choriocarcinoma was more often required among women given COCs. However, studies in the United States have since reported the very opposite (more rapid decrease of beta-human chorionic gonadotropin (β-hCG) levels post partum in COC users). After consideration of all available evidence, WHO and UKMEC now both say this is WHO 1, for any hormonal method. However, avoid use of any intrauterine methods (WHO 4) if there is frank malignancy or persistently elevated b-hCG levels because there may be an increased risk of perforation.

Carcinomas of the ovary and of the endometrium

The good news is that both cancers are definitely less frequent in COC users. Numerous studies have shown that the incidence of both is roughly halved among all users, and it is reduced to one third in long-term users; a protective effect can be detected in ex-users for up to 10 to 15 years. Suppression of ovulation in COC users and of normal mitotic activity in the endometrium is the accepted explanation of these findings.

Clinical implications

It would be reasonable for a woman known to be predisposed to either of these cancers to choose to use a CHC primarily for this protective effect.

Colorectal cancer

More than one study now suggests a significantly reduced risk for this cancer. In the RCGP study, the relative risk for current COC users in addition to those whose last use was less than 5 years earlier was 0.49, with greater protection in long-term users. However, so far the studies have not been able to show a long-term protective effect among ex-users.

Other cancers

Associations have been mooted but not confirmed.

Moreover, clinically

Women whose cancer is apparently cured by local radical surgery for neoplasia of the ovary, cervix and uterus and for malignant melanoma may all use CHCs (WHO 2).

Benefits and risks – a summary

To summarize, in the words of the RCGP study (2009), oral contraception 'was not associated with a significantly increased risk of any cancer... These

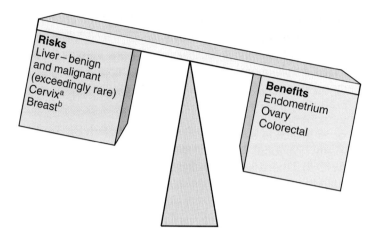

Figure 4

Cancer and COCs: a balance. [a]COC is a weak cofactor to human papillomavirus (HPV) as the oncogen. Cancer risk is minimized further by good practice (HPV vaccination, screening). [b]Small excess risk is linked to current or recent COC use, but no excess mortality is shown in ex-takers.

results suggest that, at least in this relatively healthy UK cohort, the cancer benefits associated with oral contraception outweigh the risks'. See Figure 4.

Circulatory disease and choice of COC

Venous thromboembolism

A massive UK 'Pill-scare' in 1995 could have been minimized if the data had been presented as a reduction in risk of venous thromboembolism (VTE) for women using LNG or NET Pills, in comparison with COCs containing the 'third-generation' progestogens DSG and GSD. This would have been presentationally better. It would also have been scientifically more valid because that is where the difference lies (Figure 5): the *different* progestogens are really LNG and, to a lesser extent, NET.

LNG has been shown (Figure 5) to oppose any estrogen-mediated rise in sex hormone–binding globulin (SHBG) and in high-density lipoprotein (HDL) cholesterol – and it can even lower the latter if enough is given. Somatically, it also opposes the tendency for estrogen to improve acne. It is thus unlike most other marketed progestogens, which basically allow estrogen to 'do its own thing' in a dose-dependent way. Researchers in the Netherlands and the United Kingdom have now shown that LNG when combined with EE reduces the procoagulant effects of the latter on acquired activated protein C resistance and the reduction of protein S levels. Hence, it is no longer biologically implausible that the combination of LNG with EE could (detectably but minimally) reduce the clinical risk of venous thrombosis to less than it would be with a given dose of EE alone. It looks as though DSG and GSD, and indeed most of the other progestogens used for contraception, simply fail to have that opposing action – just as they do when we actually want a greater estrogenic effect: when choosing a Pill for someone with acne, for example, where higher rather than lower SHBG levels help through binding circulating androgens.

Figure 5 (a) is thus confirmatory of clinical experience over many years, that LNG COCs are not the best choice in sebaceous disorders.

Norgestimate (NGM), the progestogen used in Cilest and Evra, the contraceptive patch, is in part metabolized to LNG. Yet both these combination products with EE seem to be clinically more estrogen dominant than Microgynon 30.

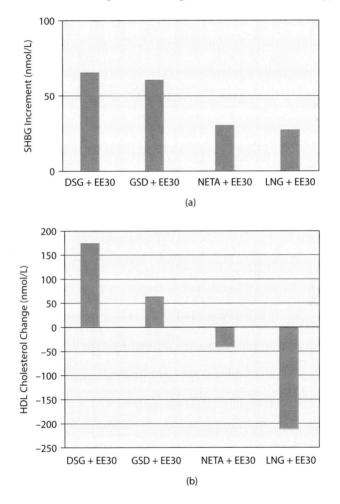

(a)

(b)

Figure 5
Prospective randomized controlled trials of four Pills: DSG 30; GSD + EE30; norethisterone acetate (NETA) + EE30; LNG + EE30. (a) Increment in SHBG. (b) Change in HDL cholesterol. (From Guillebaud J. Margaret Pyke Centre Study, 2000.)

Any beneficial effect of LNG (and NET and its pro-drugs) on VTE risk is most probably less than the epidemiology in 1995 to 1996 suggested. This is because of the influence of prescriber bias, the 'healthy-user' effect and so-called 'attrition of the susceptibles' – which led, at the time of the studies, to

- Women at lower intrinsic risk being more likely to be left using the older LNG or NET Pills – because the women with risk factors such as smoking and high body mass index (BMI) had been switched to what were thought to be the 'safer' newer products with which they were compared! Hence (the mirror image):
- Women at higher intrinsic risk tending through prescriber bias to be using DSG and GSD products, and also for new users (always an unknown quantity with respect to predisposition to VTE) to be started on these or re-started after a break from the method. These must be the non-causative explanations for the bizarre finding in WHO's VTE study of 1995 that Mercilon® containing only 20 µg EE showed an apparently greater risk of VTE than Marvelon® containing 30 µg.

Present estimates and their implications
Following a 2013 European Medicines Agency review of this VTE issue, the Medicines and Healthcare products Regulatory Agency (MHRA) cascaded to UK doctors in 2014 an important 'Alert' Letter (see https://www.cas.dh.gov.uk/ViewandAcknowledgment/ViewAlert.aspx?AlertID = 102106). In this they estimated that:

The absolute incidence for LNG/NET CHCs is *circa* 500 to 700 versus in the range 900 to 1200 per million for the third-generation progestogens DSG, GSD and also drospirenone (DSP) or CPA, the anti-androgenic progestogens that benefit acne. Using rough point estimates of 600 versus 1000 for the mean rates, this means *circa* 400 extra cases per million users per year. Assuming 1 per cent mortality for VTE, this gives (if no other risk factor) 4 per million difference in annual VTE mortality between products using LNG/NET and those not using LNG or NET or, according to a 2015 study from Nottingham, NGM (which of course is part metabolised to LNG, p. 23). *This added risk would apply if a pill-taker chooses to switch from Microgynon® to say Marvelon®, Femodene® or Dianette® but it is very similar to or less than other risks people are prepared to take (e.g. having a baby, on the roads, or in outdoor sporting activities – see Table 4 and Figure 6 plus footnotes). This small risk of switching is often acceptable for a side effect, or for acne control.*

The level of VTE risk increases with age and is likely to be increased in women with other known risk factors for VTE, such as obesity (see Table 5); and if there is an interacting disease (see p. 37).

Table 4

Comparative risks (estimated annual risks per 1 000 000)

Activity	Cases	Deaths
Having a baby, UK (all direct causes of death)		50
Having a baby (VTE)[a]	600	10
Using DSG/GSD/DSP Pill (VTE)[a]	900–1200	9–12
Using LNG/NET Pill (VTE)[a]	500–700	5–7
Non-user, non-pregnant (VTE)[a]	50–100	<1
Home accidents		30
Playing soccer		40
Road accidents (UK, 2010)		30
Parachuting (10 jumps/year)		200
Scuba diving		220
Hang-gliding		1500
Cigarette smoking (in next year if age 35 years)		1670
Death from pregnancy/childbirth in rural Africa (1990)		≥10 000

[a]VTE rates are for idiopathic cases, with no other risk factor. VTE mortality rate assumed to be 2 per cent in last edition, latest UK figures <1 per cent though higher in pregnancy: hence new estimates in right-hand column. COCs with NGM seem to share the lower risk of LNG/NET Pills, as might be expected, see p. 23.

Emphasis is on current takers and more recent data (2010). The excess mortality is acceptably small in context with the other activities shown, but is moreover so much balanced in a reproductive lifetime by the mortality benefits (e.g. in cancer; see pp. 16–22) as to make all-cause mortality in past users the same or possibly even less than for never users.

Data from Dinman BD. *JAMA* 1980; 244:1226–1228; Mills A, *et al. BMJ* 1996; 312:121; Anon. *BMJ* 1991; 302:743; Strom B. *Pharmacoepidemiology.* 2nd ed. Chichester: Wiley, 1994:57–65; www.patient.co.uk/doctor/Maternal-Mortality.htm; www.ema.europa.eu/docs/en_GB/document_library/Report/2011/05/WC500106708.pdf.

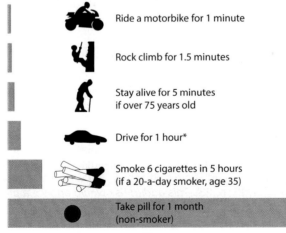

Ride a motorbike for 1 minute

Rock climb for 1.5 minutes

Stay alive for 5 minutes if over 75 years old

Drive for 1 hour*

Smoke 6 cigarettes in 5 hours (if a 20-a-day smoker, age 35)

Take pill for 1 month (non-smoker)

Time

Figure 6

*Time required to have a 1:1 000 000 risk of dying. (Adapted and updated in 2010 from Minerva, British Medical Journal, 1988.) *The estimate for car-driving is from the US National Highway Traffic Safety Administration for 1990: approximately 2 deaths per 100 million vehicle miles and assuming 50 miles driven per hour. However, later US data (2013) show a reduction; it is now 2 hours driving for 1: million risk.*

- The risk difference is tiny, but some of it at least is probably real – and therefore worth minimizing (why take any avoidable extra risk?) by the current UK policy of generally commencing with an LNG product as first line while being fully prepared to switch for symptom control on request.
- In sum, the primary reason for choosing, or changing to, a more estrogenic product, such as one containing DSG or GSD (or DSP or CPA), as the progestogen, is for the control of side effects occurring while taking a LNG or NET product.

The 2014 MHRA alert (URL as in the earlier box, p. 24) includes useful printable Annexes: 'CHC checklist for prescribers'; 'CHC user card'; and 'CHC information for women'. It is there pointed out that the risk of VTE with any CHC is higher:

- During the first year of use; and
- When re-starting use after an intake break of 4 or more weeks. (This finally destroys that widespread lay myth, that 'it's good even if the COC is suiting, to take a routine break from it after, say, 10 years'!).

Arterial diseases: acute myocardial infarction, haemorrhagic stroke and ischaemic stroke

Epidemiology, spearheaded by the WHO, has shown that the COC was not the prime cause of most of the arterial events occurring in Pill takers, both within and outside research studies.

The COC was blamed, yet arterial disease is exceptionally rare in COC takers during the reproductive years, aside from an increasing risk with age, unless they also smoke or have diabetes or hypertension. Migraine with aura is a specific, independent risk factor for ischaemic stroke.

- Acute myocardial infarction (AMI). The relative risk or OR of this condition in some studies goes up from unity (no added risk) in non-smoking controls to 10 or more in smokers also taking the COC, who indeed are in double jeopardy, because the case-fatality rate of AMI when it occurs in smokers who use the COC is also much higher.
- Haemorrhagic stroke (HS), including subarachnoid haemorrhage. The WHO and other studies have failed to show any increased risk resulting from the COC before age 35 unless there is also a risk factor such as hypertension (OR, 10) or smoking (OR, 3). The risk increases with age, and this effect is magnified by current COC use, but with no effect of past use or long-duration use.

- Ischaemic stroke (IS). Here, even in non-smokers, there is a detectable increase in the OR resulting from Pill-taking in the range of 1.5 to a maximum of 2. Much of this risk seems to be focussed within the subpopulation of women who suffer from migraine with aura (see later). The OR is 3 for hypertension and also 3 for smoking risk.
- Effects of dose/type of estrogen or progestogen? These remain uncertain and would anyway be of clinical significance only when risk factors are present, given the crucial relevance of the latter to arterial disease.

Prescribing guidelines

Current scientific evidence suggests two main prerequisites for the safe provision of COCs: a careful personal and family history with particular attention to cardiovascular risk factors, including any migraine with aura (p. 40), and a well-taken blood pressure (BP) (Hannaford P, Webb A. Evidence-guided prescribing of combined oral contraceptives: consensus statement. *Contraception* 1996;54:125–129). There should also be a baseline BMI measurement – but no other routine examinations or tests!

- Prescribers should always take a comprehensive personal and family history to exclude absolute contraindications (WHO 4) and relative contraindications (WHO 3 and 2) to the use of COCs (see pp. 28–31, 33–7).
- A personal history of definite VTE remains an absolute contraindication to any hormonal method containing EE (i.e. CHCs including Evra® or NuvaRing®), combined with any progestogen.
- The risk factors for risk of future VTE and arterial wall disease must be assessed (Tables 5 and 6).
- Note that it now appears that smoking is an independent risk factor for VTE, as well as arterial disease.
- Alone, one risk factor from either Table 5 or 6 is a relative contraindication (WHO 2 or 3 columns), unless it is particularly severe (WHO 4 column).
- Synergism means that if WHO 3 already applies, any additional risk factor moves the category to WHO 4 ('Do not use').
- Generally, however, COC use is acceptable on a WHO 3 basis when two WHO 2 factors apply.

The remarks and footnotes in Tables 5 and 6 are fundamental to Pill prescribing.

Table 5
Risk factors for venous thromboembolism (VTE)

Risk factor	Absolute contraindications	Relative contraindications		Remarks
	WHO 4	WHO 3	WHO 2	
Personal or family history (FH) of VTE or of thrombophilias	Past VTE event; or identified clotting abnormality in this person, whether hereditary or acquired.	FH of thrombosis in a parent or sibling <45 years old with or without a recognized precipitating factor (e.g. major surgery, post-partum status).	FH of VTE in a parent or sibling ≥45 years old or FH in second-degree relative.	Idiopathic VTE in a parent or sibling <45 years old is *not* now an indication for a thrombophilia screen if available – since this FH always signifies 'should use alternative FP' (WHO 3). Even a normal thrombophilia screen cannot be entirely reassuring because some predispositions are unknown.
Overweight – high BMI	BMI ≥40	BMI 30–39	BMI 25–29	Totality of data re BMI support these categories in my view, contrast UKMEC 2009. See footnotes.
Immobility	Bed-bound, with or without major surgery; or leg fractured and immobilized.	Wheelchair life, debilitating illness.	Reduced mobility for other reason.	Minor surgery such as laparoscopic sterilization is WHO 1.

Varicose veins (VVs)	Imminent VV surgery or any other VV treatment with known excess risk of VTE.	History of superficial vein thrombosis (SVT) in the lower limbs, no deep vein thrombosis.	Pulmonary embolism does not follow SVT, although past history of SVT means some caution (WHO 2) in case it may be a marker of future VTE risk. The association with VVs per se is probably coincidental.
Cigarette smoking		WHO 2 for VTE risk.	On balance, the literature now suggests a VTE risk from smoking, although less than the arterial disease risk it causes.
Age		>35 years is WHO 2, if it relates only to VTE risk.	

Notes: 1. A single risk factor in the relative contraindication columns means preference for a levonorgestrel- or norethisterone-containing Pill (British National Formulary (BNF), if any combined oral contraceptive used.

2. Beware of synergism: more than one factor in either relative contraindication column. As a working rule, two WHO 2 conditions make WHO 3; and if WHO 3 applies (e.g. BMI 30 to 39), addition of either a WHO 3 or WHO 2 (e.g. reduced mobility) condition normally means WHO 4 (do not use).

3. Acquired (non-hereditary) predispositions include positive results for antiphospholipid antibodies – definitely WHO 4 for that patient because they also increase the risk of arterial events (see Table 6).

4. Important acute VTE risk factors need to be considered in individual cases: notably, major and all leg surgery, long-haul flights and dehydration through any cause.

5. There are minor differences in the foregoing table from UKMEC, notably my (JG) more cautious categorization of BMIs higher than 25, along with clarity that a woman whose BMI is higher than 40 should avoid combined hormonal contraceptives (WHO 4).

Table 6
Risk factors for arterial disease

Risk factor	Absolute contraindications WHO 4	Relative contraindications WHO 3	WHO 2	Remarks
Family history (FH) of atherogenic lipid disorder or of arterial CVS event in sibling or parent	Identified familial hypercholesterolaemia in this person, persisting despite treatment.	FH either of known familial lipid disorder or idiopathic arterial event in parent or sibling <45 years old, and client's lipid screening result not available.	Client with previous evidence of hyperlipidaemia but responding well to treatment FH of arterial event with risk factor (e.g. smoking), in parent or sibling <45 years old, and lipid screen not available.	FH of premature (<45 years) arterial CVS disease without other risk factors, or a known atherogenic lipid disorder in a parent or sibling, indicate fasting lipid screen, where available (then check with laboratory re clinical implication of abnormal results). Despite any FH, normal lipid screen in client is reassuring, means WHO 1 (unlike thrombophilia screens).
Cigarette smoking		>15 cigarettes/day.	<15 cigarettes/day.	Cut-offs here are obviously arbitrary – see footnote 2 regarding ex-smoking.
Diabetes mellitus (DM)	Severe, long-standing or DM complications (e.g. retinopathy, renal damage, arterial disease).	Not severe/labile and no complications, young patient.		DM is always at least WHO 3 for CHCs in my (JG) view (safer options available).
Hypertension (consistently elevated BP, with properly taken measurements)	Systolic BP ≥160 mm Hg. Diastolic BP ≥95 mm Hg.	Systolic BP 140–159 mm Hg. Diastolic BP 90–94 mm Hg if essential hypertension, well controlled.	BP regularly at upper limit of normal (i.e. near to 140/90) Past history of preeclampsia (WHO 3 if also a smoker).	BP levels for categories are consistent with UKMEC but different from WHOMEC (see text).

	BMI ≥40.	BMI 30–39.	BMI 25–29.	
Overweight – high BMI				High BMI increases arterial as well as venous thromboembolic risk.
Migraine	Migraine with aura Migraine without aura if exceptionally severe lasting more than 72 hours despite optimal medication (see text).	Past migraine with aura, no recurrence in ≥5 years, terms apply (p. 42).	Migraine without aura	Relates to thrombotic stroke risk (see text for more detail; pp. 39–42).
Age >35 years	Age >35 years if a continuing smoker.	Age 35–51 years if ex-smoker (but see Note 2).	Age 35–51 years if free of all risk factors (only WHO 2, yet even safer options are available).	In all persistent smokers, age >35 years best classified as WHO 4. In ex-smokers, WHO 3 is because arterial wall damage may persist.

Notes:
1. Beware of synergism: more than one factor in either of relative contraindication columns. As a working rule, two WHO 2 conditions make WHO 3; and if WHO 3 applies (e.g. smoking ≥15/day) addition of either a WHO 3 or WHO 2 (e.g. age >35 years) condition normally means WHO 4 (as in table).
2. In continuing smokers, COC is generally stopped at age 35 years, in the United Kingdom. However, given the rapid risk reduction shown in studies of complete smoking cessation, according to UKMEC ex-smokers are classified WHO 3 only until 1 year, dropping to WHO 2 thereafter. If agreed, a LARC would usually be better still (p. 1).
3. WHO numbers also relate to use for contraception: use of COCs for medical indications such as polycystic ovarian syndrome (PCOS) often entails a different risk/benefit analysis (pp. 32–3, 38) (i.e. the extra therapeutic benefits may outweigh expected extra risks, as from a high BMI or older age, for example).
4. There are minor differences in this table from UKMEC, notably my more cautious categorization with respect to DM and smoking.

Hereditary predispositions to VTE (thrombophilias)

Genetic predispositions are rare, but when known are all classified as UKMEC 4. The most common is factor V Leiden, the genetic cause of activated protein C resistance., Even if all test results are found to be normal, however, the COC remains categorized UKMEC 3 by the family history alone (see Table 5). The woman's strong family history cannot be discounted because by no means have all the predisposing abnormalities of the complex haemostatic system yet been characterized. This is why even targeted screening by any blood test is not justifiable – the cost would be prohibitive and, in terms of what matters, which is the occurrence of actual disease events, there are just too many false-negative and false-positive results. The exception a haematologist may make is for a woman desperate to use a CHC who has a symptomatic relative with a very high-risk hereditary thrombophilia: its exclusion by testing may allow use of a CHC.

Acquired predispositions to VTE (thrombophilias)

Antiphospholipid antibodies, which increase both VTE and arterial disease risk (see Table 6, note 4) may appear in a number of connective tissue disorders, including systemic lupus erythematosus (SLE). If identified, they absolutely contraindicate COC use (WHO 4).

Which Pills are current 'best buys' for women?

- **First, all marketed Pills are 'in the frame' for prescribing.** Given the tiny possible difference in VTE mortality between the two 'generations', the woman's own choice (initially or at any later stage) of a DSG or GSD or other estrogen-dominant product rather than an LNG or NET one after (well-documented) discussion must be respected. 'The informed user should be the chooser'.
- **First-time users.** Despite what has just been said, it is generally agreed that a low-dose LNG or NET product should remain the usual first choice. This is in part because first timers will include an unknown subgroup who are VTE predisposed, VTE being a more relevant consideration than arterial disease at this age. Moreover, those Pills suit the majority and cost less. (Consider also offering the use of an everyday [ED] Pill type, which can help to reduce the chance of being a 'late restarter' after the Pill-free time – see later.)
- **In the presence of a single WHO 2 or 3 risk factor for venous thrombosis.** The Summary of Product Characteristics (SPCs) for COCs states that DSG/GSD products are contraindicated. However, if there is a clear therapeutic indication for the COC, such as PCOS in a woman with moderately severe acne, a different risk/benefit balance may apply. Extra therapeutic benefits from a more estrogenic product may be judged to outweigh (on a WHO 3 basis) any expected extra

risks because, for example, the woman has a BMI of 35. Relevant choices might be Marvelon 30, Yasmin or Dianette – or maybe even better, now, Daylette (p. 62). These probably all share the same (estrogen-dominant) category – but in my view only because they lack LNG, with its apparent ability to antagonize effects of EE, whether unwanted (prothrombotic) or wanted (e.g. SHBG increase).

- **Women with a single definite arterial risk factor (see Table 6) (e.g. smokers or diabetic patients)** – after a number of years of VTE-free use or if the COC is used at all by healthy women older than 35 years. As we have seen, in pre-menopausal women, AMI is almost exclusively a disease of smokers. However, the hazard is higher when such risk factors are present (the RCGP's relative risk estimate for AMI was 20.8 for smoking Pill takers!); it increases with age, and the case-fatality rate for AMI in Pill takers is also higher. Some studies (but not others) suggest that DSG/GSD Pills may have relative advantages for arterial wall disease. Therefore, for such higher-risk women, or for women without any such risk factors but who are older, 35 through to approximately 51 years old (the average of the menopause), using a 20-µg DSG or GSD product or the natural estrogen-containing Pills Zoely or Qlaira may be proposed. Any advantages in so doing are far from established, and changing to a different method altogether would usually be a better course.
- **Finally, the primary reason for ever-changing COC brands is the control of side effects, for the woman's quality of life.** If, for any indication, she moves to using a product not containing LNG or NET, it should be documented that she accepts a possible tiny increase in the risk of VTE. See Table 4 and Figure 6 on p. 25.

Eligibility criteria for COCs

Absolute contraindications to COCs or other CHCs, including NuvaRing and Evra

As already mentioned, all lists of absolute or relative contraindications in this book are based on UKMEC, with a very few differences based on the author's judgement of the evidence. Compare with the Faculty Guidance document First Prescription of Combined Oral Contraception, at www.fsrh. org: several important conditions in the following list (e.g. porphyria, hyper-triglyceridaemia, pemphigoid gestationis and idiopathic intracranial hyper-tension) are not mentioned in relation to the COC there, or in UKMEC 2009.

All conditions in this first list are WHO 4 for the COC. However, as shown later, for the same conditions progestogen-only Pills (POPs), including the DSG POP, and other progestogen-only methods, are in most cases classi-fied no higher than WHO 2.

1. **Past or present circulatory disease.**
   - Any past proven arterial or venous thrombosis.
   - Established ischaemic heart disease or angina or coronary arteritis (current Kawasaki disease – past history is WHO 3 or 2, depending on completeness of recovery). Also significant peripheral vascular disease.
   - Multiple risk factors for venous or arterial disease.
   - Severe single factors can also be enough for the WHO 4 category (see Tables 5 and 6):
     - BMI > 40.
     - BP >160/>95 mm Hg.
     - Diabetes with tissue damage.
   - Atherogenic lipid disorders (some not all, a complex issue, take advice from an expert).
   - Known prothrombotic states (i.e. any of foregoing congenital or acquired thrombophilias, including SLE if antiphospholipid antibodies are positive or unknown). Secondary Raynaud's phenomenon indicates testing for these:
     - From at least 2 (preferably 4) weeks before until 2 weeks after mobilization following elective major surgery (do not demand that the COC be stopped for minor surgery such as brief laparoscopy with minimal post-operative immobilization) and almost all leg surgery (e.g. operative arthroscopy of knee, or for varicose veins).
     - During leg immobilization (e.g. after fracture).
   - Migraine with aura (described on pp. 39–42).
   - Definite aura without a headache following.
   - Past ischaemic stroke, transient ischaemic attacks (TIAs).
   - Past cerebral haemorrhage.
   - Pulmonary hypertension, any cause.
   - Structural heart disease (e.g. valvular heart disease or shunts or septal defects) is WHO 4 if there is an added arterial or venous thromboembolic risk (persisting, if there has been surgery). Always discuss this with the cardiologist – could be WHO 3, especially if the patient is always anticoagulated. Even better choices (WHO 2 or 1) in most of these conditions would be the DSG POP or any LARC (caution re vasovagal risk at insertion of IUCs).
   - Important WHO 4 examples, for CHCs:
     - Atrial fibrillation or flutter whether sustained or paroxysmal – or not current but high risk (e.g. mitral stenosis).
     - Cyanotic heart disease.
     - Any dilated cardiomyopathy; but this is classified as only WHO 2 when in full remission after a past history of any type (including pregnancy cardiomyopathy).
   - In other structural heart conditions, if there is little or no direct or indirect risk of thromboembolism (this being the crucial point to check with the cardiologist), the COC is usable (WHO 3 or 2) For more on cardiac disease, see http://www.fsrh.org/pdfs/ CEUGuidanceContraceptiveChoicesWomenCardiacDisease.pdf.

2. **Liver.**
   - Liver adenoma, carcinoma.
   - Active liver cell disease, whenever liver function tests are currently significantly abnormal, including infiltrations, severe chronic hepatitis B and C, and cirrhosis (although UKMEC allows WHO 1 for cirrhosis that is *compensated*).
   - Past Pill-related cholestatic jaundice; if this was only in pregnancy and never with the COC, this can be classified WHO 2. (Contrast UKMEC, permitting WHO 3, not WHO 4 as I advise here, if the attack was Pill related.)
   - During any acute viral hepatitis, but COCs may be resumed once liver function test results have become normal (and a .clinical test of two units of alcohol consumption is tolerated).
   - Dubin-Johnson and Rotor syndromes are rare benign genetic disorders of hepatic secretion. COCs, like pregnancy, can cause overt jaundice (Gilbert's disease is WHO 2).
3. **History of serious condition affected by sex steroids or related to previous COC use.**
   - SLE – suggestion that COCs may worsen the condition, but there is thrombotic risk anyway.
   - COC-induced hypertension.
   - Pancreatitis from hypertriglyceridaemia.
   - Pemphigoid gestationis.
   - Chorea.
   - Stevens-Johnson syndrome (erythema multiforme), if COC-associated.
   - Haemolytic uraemic syndrome (HUS) and thrombotic thrombocytopenic purpura (TTP); HUS in past is WHO 2.
4. **Pregnancy.**
5. **Estrogen-dependent neoplasms.**
   - Breast cancer.
   - Past breast biopsy showing pre-malignant epithelial atypia.
6. **Miscellaneous.**
   - Allergy to any COC constituent.
   - Past idiopathic intracranial hypertension.
   - Specific to Yasmin (or Daylette®): avoid, because of the unique spironolactone-like effects of drospirenone, in anyone at risk of high potassium levels (including severe renal insufficiency, hepatic dysfunction and treatment with potassium-sparing diuretics).
   - Sturge-Weber syndrome (thrombotic stroke risk).
   - Post-partum status for 6 weeks if breastfeeding (according to UKMEC, but is anyway redundant for contraception).
7. **Woman's anxiety about COC safety unrelieved by counselling.**

Note that several of the items in this list (e.g. 4, 5 and 7) are not necessarily permanent contraindications. Moreover, many women over the years have been unnecessarily deprived of COCs for reasons now believed to have no link, such as thrush or otosclerosis; or that would have positively benefited from the method, such as secondary amenorrhoea with hypo-estrogenism.

Relative contraindications to COCs

The following list provides the relative contraindications to COCs, WHO 2 or 3, signifying that the COC method is usable in context with:

- The benefit/risk evaluation for that individual.
- The acceptability or otherwise of alternatives.
- Sometimes with special advice (e.g. in migraine, to report a change of symptomatology) or monitoring.
- In patients with excess risk of venous thrombosis (e.g. wheelchair life – WHO 3 – see Table 5), if the Pill is used at all for contraception, it should perhaps be a LNG/NET variety.

For relative contraindications, please read the following box in conjunction with Tables 5 and 6, which deal with the most common issues (e.g. smoking, obesity and hypertension).

Unless otherwise stated below, COCs (like all CHCs of course) are WHO 2:

Relative contraindications
- Risk factors for arterial or venous disease (see Tables 5 and 6). These are WHO 2, sometimes 3 (e.g. in my view any BMI higher than 30 is at least WHO 3): provided that only one is present and that not of such severity as to justify WHO 4.
  - HUS (see earlier): in past history may be WHO 2 if complete recovery and not Pill associated (e.g. past *Escherichia coli* O157 infection being the established cause of past attack of HUS)
  - Diabetes (minimum category being WHO 3), hypertensive disease and migraine all deserve separate discussion (see later)
  - Post-partum status during the first 3 weeks (WHO 3 through the post-delivery VTE risk, but negligible fertility anyway)
- Most chronic congenital or acquired systemic diseases (see later) are WHO 2.
- Risk of altitude illness is not more probable because a climber is on COC; but if it occurs, in its most severe forms, venous or arterial thromboembolism or patchy pulmonary hypertension is known to occur, which would contraindicate the method.
- Hence, women climbing to more than 4500 m should be informed that the COC may increase the thrombotic component of altitude illness if that were to occur (WHO 3) – and also the risk of VTE. The COC would be WHO 3, but could be only WHO 2 in many healthy trekkers who intend always to follow the maxim 'climb high but sleep low'. More details are in *BMJ* 2003;326:915–919; *BMJ* 2011; 343:d4943 and in Faculty Guidance (URL on p. 13).

- Sex steroid–dependent cancer in prolonged remission (WHO 3) – prolonged is defined as after 5 years by UKMEC: prime example is breast cancer.
- If a young (<40 years of age) first-degree relative has breast cancer or the woman herself has benign breast disease (WHO 2, although UKMEC says WHO 1). Being a known carrier of one of the *BRCA* genes is WHO 3 (p. 19).
- Malignant melanoma has been shown to be unrelated, so is WHO 2 for the Pill.
- During the monitoring of abnormal cervical smears (WHO 2).
- During and after definitive treatment for CIN (WHO 2).
- Oligo/amenorrhoea (COCs may be prescribed, after investigation – may be WHO 1, use unrestricted, if the purpose is to supply estrogen in a woman needing contraception or to control the symptoms of PCOS).
- Hyperprolactinaemia is WHO 3, but only for patients who are on specialist drug treatment and with close supervision.
- Sickle cell trait is WHO 1, but homozygous sickle cell disease is WHO 2 (although DMPA is preferred for this).
- Inflammatory bowel disease is WHO 2, or (my view) WHO 3 if severe, because of known VTE risk in exacerbations (WHO 4; i.e., stop COC if hospitalized). Absorption of the COC may be reduced in Crohn's disease of the small bowel, but only if it is severe with evidence of malabsorption.
- Acute porphyria is WHO 3 in my view because COCs can precipitate a first attack (and 1 per cent of attacks are fatal). Other porphyrias are WHO 2, but a non-hormone method is usually preferable.
- Gallstones: symptomatic, medically treated (WHO 3, but WHO 2 if are an incidental finding; or after cholecystectomy).
- Very severe depression, if there is a history of its seemingly being exacerbated by COCs (but unwanted pregnancies can be very depressing! – and evidence supports that COCs do not cause depression).
- Diseases that require long-term treatment with enzyme-inducing drugs are WHO 3 (COC is usable [see later] – but alternative contraception is preferred).
- Undiagnosed genital tract bleeding (WHO 3 until diagnosed and as necessary treated).

Intercurrent diseases

It is impossible for the foregoing lists to include every known disease that may have a bearing (i.e. WHO 4, 3 or 2) on COC prescription, and for many the data are unavailable.

Therefore, what principles may be applied?

First, is there summation? Are there disease effects that are additive to known adverse effects of CHCs generally or the COC in particular, or (less commonly) progestogen-only methods?

In particular, does the condition or risk factor:
1. Increase the risk of arterial or venous thrombosis, anywhere? This includes consideration of:
    *   Restricted mobility even if the disease is otherwise unrelated to thrombosis risk.
    *   Atrial fibrillation with its known risk of systemic embolism.
2. Predispose to arterial wall disease or hypertension?
3. Adversely affect liver function?
4. Require treatment with an interacting drug (e.g. an enzyme-inducer drug [EID]?)

If none of items 1 to 4 apply, the condition can usually be considered as at most WHO 2 for any of the CHCs.
If any do apply, CHC use will be either WHO 4 or WHO 3.
Note: WHO 3 always implies 'an alternative preferable'.
Are the CHCs being given as therapy, not contraception alone?
The added non-contraceptive benefit (from the CHC as therapy) and, in some diseases, the avoidance of extra risk from pregnancy may then be held to justify some added risk affecting the woman (i.e. the risk/benefit difference could be judged similar to normal CHC taking). Common examples are:
*   PCOS + acne yet a high BMI, or
*   Heavy menstrual bleeding with high BMI (and she declines an LNG-IUS or surgery).

Yet, the added risk *per se* remains the same as if the CHC was not being used thus, as treatment. Hence, record that this was discussed and fully accepted by the patient, along with consideration of other reliable choices that are free of EE and therefore of added thrombotic risk (e.g. the desogestrel POP, implants, IUDs and the IUS).

Diabetes mellitus

In general, and whether type 1 or type 2 DM, this is generally a WHO 3 condition for CHCs (JG), even when there is no known overt diabetic tissue damage (see Table 6 – and contrast UKMEC, which classes well-controlled DM as WHO 2).

DMPA is also WHO 3 (JG) in DM, given its SPC that reports a 15 to 20 per cent reduction in HDL-cholesterol.

So the POP (often a DSG POP), an implant, a modern copper IUD, or a LNG-IUS are all definitely preferred to any of the CHCs. These can all be started right after coitarche in young diabetic patients. If CHCs are, reluctantly, used, it should be for patients with no known arteriopathy, retinopathy, neuropathy or renal damage, or any added circulatory risk factor such as obesity or smoking (all of which mean WHO 4) – and in my view only if the duration of the disease has been less than 20 years. Moreover, the natural estradiol-containing Zoely or Qlaira may be safer (less prothrombotic, pp. 63–4) than CHC products that give an ultra-low dose of EE (i.e. NuvaRing and the 20-μg COCs of Table 2). Even these CHCs should be used with due caution (WHO 3), and with the plan to switch to an estrogen-free method whenever acceptable; and often sterilization after childbearing is complete.

Hypertension

Hypertension is an important risk factor for both heart disease and stroke (see Table 6).

- In most women on COCs, there is a slight increase in both systolic and diastolic BP within the normotensive range: less than 1 per cent of women become clinically hypertensive with modern low doses, but the rate increases with age and duration of use. Above 140/90 mm Hg, this is classified as WHO 3; but if BP is repeatedly higher than 160/95 (either the systolic or diastolic figure), I agree with UKMEC that the method should be stopped; and even if it then normalizes, this Pill-induced hypertension means WHO 4 for the future.
- Past severe pregnancy-induced hypertension does not predispose to hypertension during COC use, but even without this it is a risk factor for myocardial infarction (WHO 2) – markedly so if the women also smokes (WHO 3).
- Essential hypertension (not COC related), when well controlled on drugs, is WHO 3 (i.e. the COC is usable, but not ideal if an effective alternative is acceptable).

Migraine

Like hypertension, this condition is of critical relevance both at the first prescription and during the follow-up for all users of combined hormonal contraception (CHC).

Migraines can be defined by the answers to the following questions:
During the last 3 months did you have the following with your headaches?
1. You felt nauseated or sick in your stomach.
2. You were bothered by light a lot more than when you don't have headache.

Migraine and stroke risk

- Studies have shown an increased risk of ischaemic stroke if there is migraine with aura or COC-use, and if combined, 'summation' of risk.
- There is good evidence of exacerbation of risk by arterial risk factors, including smoking and increasing age beyond 35 years.
- The presence of aura before (or sometimes even **without**) the headache is the main marker of risk of ischaemic stroke (WHO 4). However, it seems increasingly likely that there is no significantly increased risk through having migraine without aura – although for the present this is still classified as WHO 2. Given that the 1-year prevalence of any migraine in women has been shown to be as high as 18 per cent, it is crucial to identify the important subgroup with aura (1-year prevalence about 5 per cent).

Migraine with aura

- Taking this crucial history starts by establishing the timing: neurological symptoms of aura begin before the headache itself, and typically last around 20 to 30 minutes (maximum 60 minutes) and stop before the headache (which may be very mild). Headache may start as aura is resolving, or there may be a gap of up to 1 hour.

- Visual symptoms occur in 99 per cent of true auras and hence should be asked about first.
- These auras are typically bright and affect part of the field of vision, on the same side in both eyes (homonymous hemianopia).
- Fortification spectra are often described, typically a bright scintillating zigzag line gradually enlarging from a bright centre on one side, to form a convex C-shape surrounding the area of lost vision (which is a bright scotoma).
- Sensory symptoms are confirmatory of aura, occurring in around one third of cases and rarely in the absence of visual aura. Typically, they come as 'pins and needles' (paraesthesia) spreading up one arm or one side of the face or the tongue; the leg is rarely affected. They are positive symptoms – not loss of function.
- Disturbance of speech may also occur, in the form of dysphasia.

Note the absence in the foregoing box of the symptoms that occur during headache itself (photophobia or, e.g., generalized blurring or 'flashing lights'). Moreover, aura symptoms should not be confused with premonitory symptoms, such as food cravings, excessive lethargy, extra sensitivity to light and sound, occurring a day or so before any migraine (i.e. with or without aura) and often continuing into the headache.

Clinical implications

- Ask the woman to describe a typical attack from the very beginning, including any symptoms before a headache. Listen to what she says, but at the same time watch her carefully.
- A most useful sign that what she describes is likely to be true aura is if she waves her hand on one or other side of her own head and draws something like a zigzag line in the air.

In summary, aura has three main features:
- Characteristic timing: onset before (headache) and duration up to 1 hour and resolution before or with onset of headache.
- Symptoms visual (99 per cent).
- Description visible (using a hand).

Migraine-related absolute contraindications (WHO 4) to starting or continuing the COC or any CHC
- Migraine with aura or aura alone with no following headache. The artificial estrogen of the COC is what needs to be avoided (or stopped, at once and forever) to minimize the additional risk of a thrombotic stroke.
- Migraine attack without aura that is exceptionally severe in a woman who has just started taking a CHC and lasting more than 72 hours despite optimal medication needs evaluation; it could be WHO 3 in an established COC user with migraine without aura, once fully assessed.
- All migraines treated with ergot derivatives because of their vasoconstrictor actions. (Triptans are much preferred for most women.)

Note that in all the foregoing circumstances, any of the progestogen-only (i.e. estrogen-free) hormonal methods may be offered immediately. Similar headaches may continue, but now without the potential added risk from pro-thrombotic effects of EE.

Particularly useful choices are the POP (a DSG POP in the young), an implant, the LNG-IUS, or a modern copper IUD (all WHO 1 in my view, although strangely WHOMEC and UKMEC both classify the first three as WHO 2).

> **WHO 3: The COC is usable with caution and close supervision**
> - Erring probably on the side of caution (JG), this means migraine without aura (common or simple migraine) where there are also important risk factor(s) for ischaemic stroke present. A good example is heavy smoking, which itself is a significant risk factor for ischaemic stroke.
> - Second, a clear past history of typical migraine with aura more than 5 years earlier or only during pregnancy, with no recurrence, may be regarded as WHO 3. COCs may be given a trial, with counselling and regular supervision, along with a specific warning that the onset of definite aura (carefully explained) means that the user should
>   - Stop the Pill immediately.
>   - Use alternative contraception.
>   - Seek medical advice as soon as possible.

Migraine: relative contraindications for the COC

> **WHO 2: The COC is certainly 'broadly useable' in the following cases**
> - Migraine without aura, and also without any arterial risk factor from Table 6, even if it is the woman's first ever attack occurring while taking the COC (this is a change from previous advice). Note that if these (or indeed other 'ordinary' headaches) occur only or mainly in the Pill-free interval (PFI), tricycling or continuous use of the COC may help.
> - Use of a triptan drug in the absence of any other contraindicating factors.

Differential diagnoses

It may be difficult to distinguish relatively common, migraine-associated focal neurological symptoms from rare organic episodes – true TIAs. TIAs are more sudden in onset than migraine aura, and although they usually last less than an hour, they often include weakness or paralysis of the face, arm or leg, which is not typical in migraine. On suspicion, these of course mean the same in practice (i.e. WHO 4) – stop the Pill immediately. If an organic episode is a possibility, hospital investigation should also follow.

The following features are not typical of migraine

- Focal epilepsy, severe acute vertigo, hemiparesis, ataxia, aphasia or unilateral tinnitus.
- A severe unexplained drop attack or collapse.
- Monocular blindness (black scotoma) – this could rarely be a retinal vascular event or a symptom of TIA (amaurosis fugax).

- Progressive or persistent neurological symptoms (migraine is episodic, with a refractory period, hence complete freedom from symptoms between attacks). Daily headaches are not migraine.

The 'Pill-free interval' and its implications for COC prescribing and maintenance of efficacy

Because no contraceptive is being taken during the PFI, it has important efficacy implications (Figure 7). Biochemical and ultrasound data obtained at the Margaret Pyke Centre (MPC) and elsewhere demonstrate return of significant pituitary and ovarian follicular activity during the PFI in about 20 per cent of cases – to a marked extent in some – but even in these cases, renewed Pill taking after no more than a 7-day PFI restores ovarian quiescence. However, these data make it clear that any lengthening of the PFI beyond 7 days is likely to lead to breakthrough ovulation. Lengthening of the PFI may be caused either side of the 'horseshoe' in Figure 7 (i.e. from omissions, malabsorption as from vomiting, or enzyme-inducing drug interactions that involve Pills either at the start or at the end of a packet).

All COC users generally think the 'worst' Pills to miss are in the middle of a packet (i.e. they use the wrong analogy with the middle of a normal cycle).

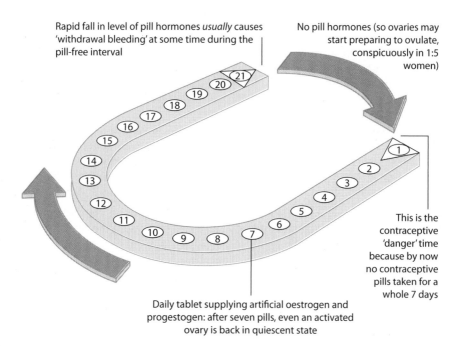

Rapid fall in level of pill hormones *usually* causes 'withdrawal bleeding' at some time during the pill-free interval

No pill hormones (so ovaries may start preparing to ovulate, conspicuously in 1:5 women)

This is the contraceptive 'danger' time because by now no contraceptive pills taken for a whole 7 days

Daily tablet supplying artificial oestrogen and progestogen: after seven pills, even an activated ovary is back in quiescent state

Figure 7
'Horseshoe' analogy to explain the 21-day cycle. Omission of tablets either side of the gap in the horseshoe lengthens the 'contraception-losing interval' (see text).

Indeed, the 'worst Pills', actually the first two in any pack, are not seen by most COC takers as even being 'missed Pills'! Starting the next pack late – just after the falsely reassuring withdrawal bleeding – does not trigger them even to seek advice about maintaining their contraception – unless they have been properly taught. What ought to be explained, but too often is not, is the contraception-weakening effect of the PFI. It helps to make a *horseshoe* with one's hand (see Figure 7). Then say: *'It's pretty simple, after 7 days without any pills your ovary may already have begun to 'wake up', getting ready to release an egg, so of course it is 'very bad news' to be late restarting the next pack'. Each woman should leave the COC consultation with a simple mantra in her head: 'I must never be a late restarter... I must never be a late restarter'...* and understand what to do if she is (see the box on p. 45).

Mobile phones. Almost all Pill takers in the United Kingdom have one of these, with a calendar function. Teaching about the COC, indeed all CHCs, should now include 'set your mobile to remind you every 28 days to commence a new pack (or patch, or ring)'. This is much more important for most women than being reminded every 24 hours to take one of the 21 active tablets. Dedicated apps are also available; 28-day packaging can help, by increasing the chance of the user noticing during her PFI that she needs a new supply of her method.

A population of current Pill users was studied after the end of a routine PFI (Smith S, *et al. Contraception* 1986;34:513–522). The study showed that if only 14 or even as few as 7 Pills were then taken, no fertile ovulation occurred after 7 Pills were subsequently missed. This and other work may be summarized as follows:

- Seven consecutive Pills are enough 'to shut the door' on the ovaries (therefore Pills 8 to 21, or longer during tricycling, simply 'keep the door shut').
- Seven Pills can be omitted without ovulation, as indeed is regularly the case in the PFI.
- More than seven Pills missed (in total) risks ovulation.

Clinical implications

The duration of clinicians' uncertainty about what advice to give women who have missed tablets is incredible: it is 50 years since the COC was first marketed in the United Kingdom! Based on another review of the evidence, the UK MHRA at last (2011) produced what I consider acceptable advice for 'missed Pills'.

Given the known marked individual variation in ovarian responses, which have much greater significance for efficacy than the Pill dose taken, I have always favoured instructions that err on the side of caution; so long as they are evidence based, as summarized in Figure 7 and, above all, conveyed as simply as can be.

What follows is unchanged from what I have regularly recommended in previous editions. The definition of a 'missed Pill' is '24 hours late' (in line with WHO, although the SPCs of most manufacturers continue to say 12 hours). There are then just four bullet points to the advice that I continue to recommend:

- 'ONE tablet missed, for up to 24 hours': aside from taking the delayed Pill as soon as remembered and the next one on time, no special action is needed. This applies up to the time that two tablets would need to be taken at once.
- 'MORE THAN ONE tablet missed' (i.e. anything more than 24 hours elapsed since an active Pill should have been taken, and a second tablet also late by one or maybe many more hours): Use CONDOMS as well, for the next 7 days.

Plus:

- If this happened in the third active Pill week, at the end of the pack RUN ON to the next pack (skipping seven placebos if present).
- In the first Pill week, with sexual exposure since the last pack ended, EMERGENCY CONTRACEPTION (EC) is recommended IF:
  - The user is a 'late restarter' by more than 2 days (>9-day PFI); *or*
  - More than two Pills are missed in the first week; *or*
- She had a more than 9 day PFI through missed Pills at the end of the last pack.

Hormonal EC usually by LNG EC, see pp. 141–2, should be followed, next day, by taking the appropriate day's tablet.

Figure 8 presents the same advice in a flowchart for users. In both the box and Figure 8, note my preference for the wording 'more than one Pill missed' rather than the MHRA's 'two or more Pills missed'. These are not synonymous in practice. The wording used here is both

- More cautious (as I favour: to ensure the least chance of failure with omissions of any of the crucial Pills 1 to 7); and
- Makes it completely clear that a woman who is late with one tablet by (say) 36 hours and a second one also, but so far by only 12 hours, should begin to use condoms for any sex.

Almost all current and past advice is overly cautious for missed Pills later than the first week. In the third week, if a Pill user omits three to four Pills and does follow the instruction to miss her next routine PFI by running on to the next pack, she will be even less likely to ovulate than usual.

Every time you miss any one pill (late by up to 24 hours):

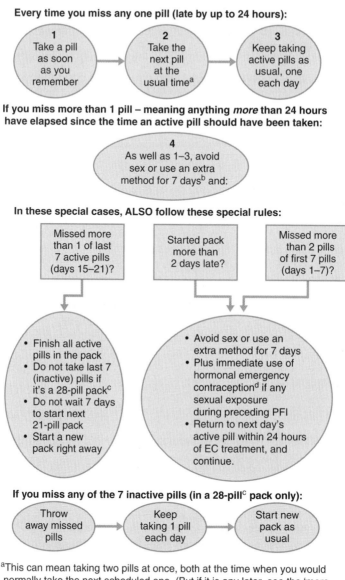

1
Take a pill as soon as you remember

2
Take the next pill at the usual time[a]

3
Keep taking active pills as usual, one each day

If you miss more than 1 pill – meaning anything *more* than 24 hours have elapsed since the time an active pill should have been taken:

4
As well as 1–3, avoid sex or use an extra method for 7 days[b] and:

In these special cases, ALSO follow these special rules:

Missed more than 1 of last 7 active pills (days 15–21)?

Started pack more than 2 days late?

Missed more than 2 pills of first 7 pills (days 1–7)?

- Finish all active pills in the pack
- Do not take last 7 (inactive) pills if it's a 28-pill pack[c]
- Do not wait 7 days to start next 21-pill pack
- Start a new pack right away

- Avoid sex or use an extra method for 7 days
- Plus immediate use of hormonal emergency contraception[d] if any sexual exposure during preceding PFI
- Return to next day's active pill within 24 hours of EC treatment, and continue.

If you miss any of the 7 inactive pills (in a 28-pill[c] pack only):

Throw away missed pills

Keep taking 1 pill each day

Start new pack as usual

[a]This can mean taking two pills at once, both at the time when you would normally take the next scheduled one. (But if it is any later, see the 'more than 1 pill' advice.)

[b]9 days for Qlaira—*plus* see text.

[c]28-pill (ED) packs can obviously help some pill-takers not to forget to restart after each PFI (the contraception-losing interval) (see text). Even with triphasic pills, you should go straight to (the first phase of) the same brand. You may bleed a bit but you will still strengthen your contraception.

[d]LNG EC is usually preferred to UPA EC in 'missed-pills', see pp. 141–2.

Figure 8
Advice for missed Pills. (Regarding Pill days 8 to 14, see p. 47).

In the second week, the seven or more Pills she has taken will have made her ovary quiescent after the previous PFI, so three to four tablets missed should not be enough to allow ovulation. Hence, the advice to use condoms for 7 days is highly fail-safe: if a woman worries that it was not followed, EC would be needed only if the history suggests seriously erratic Pill taking, earlier, as well.

If 28-day packs are used (e.g. Microgynon ED, which usefully helps to avoid risky 'late restarts'), the user must learn which are the dummy 'reminder' tablets. If she misses some of the last seven (yellow) active Pills, she must be taught to omit all the (white) placebos.

After Pill-taking errors or severe vomiting or short-term use of an enzyme-inducer drug (see later), all women should be asked to report back if they have no withdrawal bleeding in the next PFI.

Vomiting and diarrhoea

If vomiting began over 2 hours after a Pill was taken, it can be assumed to have been absorbed. Otherwise, follow the advice in the box on page 48 or Figure 8, according to the number and timing of the tablets deemed to have been missed. Diarrhoea alone is not a problem, unless it is of cholera-like severity.

Previous COC failure

Women who have had a previous COC failure may claim perfect compliance or perhaps admit to omission of no more than one Pill. Either way, as surveys show, most women miss a tablet quite frequently yet rarely conceive, so genuine Pill failure tells us more about the individual's physiology than her memory. She is likely to be a member of that one fifth of the population whose ovaries show above-average return to activity in the PFI. Such women may well be advised to choose a LARC, but they could also use one of the extended regimens of Pill taking (see later).

Once it has been appreciated that the Achilles' heel of the COC is the PFI, the COC can always be made 'stronger' as a contraceptive, by eliminating and/or shortening the PFI through numerous variations on the tricycling theme depicted in Figure 9. Alternatively, for women who still wish to 'see'

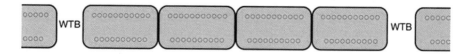

Figure 9
Tricycling. Note the use of monophasic packs, as in Seasonale® which equates to four packs in a row. Duration of the Pill-free interval may also, preferably, be shortened from 7 to 4 days, or of course to 0 days in 365/365 combined oral contraceptive regimens (see text). WTB, withdrawal bleeding.

monthly bleeds (p. 48), greater efficacy can come through a shortened PFI, as in Daylette® or Zoely® (pp. 62, 64).

Regimens for extended COC taking

For many years, in the short term, the gap between packets of monophasic brands has often been omitted at the woman's choice, to avoid a 'period' on special occasions and on holidays.

This practice is approved and appears in most SPCs and PILs. Users of phasic Pills who wish to postpone withdrawal bleeding must use the final phase of a spare packet, or Pills from an equivalent formulation (e.g. Microgynon 30 immediately after the last tablet of Logynon).

Why have any PFIs at all?

The Pill-free week does promote a withdrawal bleeding episode, which some women prefer and find reassuring. Indeed, if it does not occur as expected in two successive cycles, it is standard teaching to rule out pregnancy by using a sensitive urine hCG test. However, this hormone-withdrawal bleeding is irrelevant to maintaining health. So there is another group of women who are delighted not to have it – and moreover may wish to obtain the other advantages listed in the 'extended use' box (later) by simply omitting most or all the PFIs, as a long-term option (see Figure 9).

Note that no form of long-term extended use is as yet (2015) licensed in the United Kingdom. However, in the United States, Seasonale® is a dedicated tricycle-type packaging that provides four packets of the formulation of Microgynon/Ovranette in a row, followed by a 7-day Pill-free week, such that the user has bleeding every 3 months (i.e. seasonally!). This variant requires 16 packets a year, as compared with the usual 13 packs. Seasonique® is similar, with added estrogen-only during the 3-monthly PFI of 7 days. Because 30-µg EE Pills are used by these tricycling brands, the annual ingested dose is obviously greater than in traditional 21/28 regimens. Therefore, they cannot be expected to reduce the risks of major or minor side effects – although the prospective user may be advised that there is no evidence that these Pills will significantly increase them, either.

Since 2003, mainly in America (North and South) there have been a number of promising RCTs of lower doses (usually 20 µg EE) comparing absolutely continuous (365/365) Pill taking with the traditional method. These have demonstrated acceptable bleeding patterns for most (not all) users – including, in Leslie Miller's study *Obstet Gynecol* 2003;101:653–661, no bleeding at all in 72 per cent of continuing users at 9 to 10 months (though there was a high drop-out rate). Unlike tricycling, using 20-µg Pills these regimens entail taking less EE in a year than any 30-µg COC taken in the traditional 21/28 way (see the later box).

Continuous low-dose Pills seem to work best, and based on Miller's work, continuous EE 20 μg/LNG 90 μg has arrived on some markets as Lybrel® (or Anya®) since 2008. Edelman *et al. Obstet Gynecol* 2006;107:657–665, in an RCT of LNG versus NET formulations, found that sustained use of a Pill equivalent to the Loestrin 20 in the United Kingdom was better than the EE 20 μg with LNG product for producing amenorrhoea. Therefore, pending marketing of a dedicated product in the United Kingdom – something many prescribers and users would welcome – women who wish to do so may try taking Loestrin 20 continuously – on an unlicensed basis (p. 165). Although not yet formally tested, other 20-μg COCs may also be used, similarly, always with warning that light, usually, but unpredictable spotting occurs – especially early on. Microgynon 30 has also been evaluated in an RCT at the MPC, but 30-μg EE brands are not favoured (JG) because of the increased annual EE dose (10950 ug).

Some potential advantages of extended (365/365) COC regimens (e.g. using Loestrin 20)

- More convenient and the option, maybe, if oligo-amenorrhoea is achieved, of more days available for sex!
- Cheaper; less sanitary protection is needed: because despite more breakthrough bleeding (BTB) or spotting, there are many fewer *scheduled* bleeding days (i.e. normally, 13 times a year).
- Good wherever there is suspicion of decreased efficacy.
- Much greater margin for Pill-taking errors: up to 7 pills are missable with no more conception risk than there is 13 times a year in normal 21/7 regimens!
- Less confusing 'rules': indeed, missed-Pill advice (up to 7 tablets) boils down to one instruction, simply 'return to regular Pill-taking'!
- Useful option in long-term enzyme-inducer therapy (p. 52).
- Lower annual dose of EE if 20 μg for all 365 days (7300 μg) than 30 μg taken 21/28 (8190 μg).
- Maintained or likely improved non-contraceptive benefits. Already shown:
  - Fewer cyclical symptoms (especially fewer headaches in the PFI and less COC-related premenstrual syndrome [PMS] reported).
  - No heavy or painful COC-withdrawal bleeding.
- Less anaemia.
  Needing confirmation epidemiologically:
  - Cancer prevention (*possibility* it even improves on pp. 21–2).
  - Endometriosis – expected to be particularly good for this (both as to prevention and for maintenance therapy).
  - In epilepsy, sustained hormone levels may reduce seizure frequency.

With slight modification, most of these advantages are also to be expected, if the woman prefers to bleed periodically by tricycling (Figure 9).

Unacceptable bleeding with extended COC use – the 'tailored pill'

For the user of either 365/365 or any tricycling regimen, a method exists of dealing with undesired bleeding which is usually effective. The user is advised, in advance, that if the duration of any such bleeding is unacceptable (e.g. >4 days), she can at any time (so long as >7 Pills have been taken consecutively) simply let the bleeding trigger her to take a break from Pill taking – for 4 days. This is empowering (Sisters doing it for themselves. *J Fam Plann Reprod Health Care* 2009;35:71–2). It probably works through being what could be termed a pharmacological curettage, after which with resumed Pill taking oligo-amenorrhoea often returns and the need for such bleeding-triggered breaks usually diminishes with time.

Drug interactions

Interacting drugs can reduce the efficacy of COCs by induction of liver enzymes, which leads to increased elimination of both estrogen and progestogen (Figure 10). This effect can as much as halve blood levels of both hormones, be maintained after cessation for a remarkable 28 days and is clinically important.

Do antibiotics matter anymore?

In 2010, the WHO reviewed the evidence relating to the recirculation of EE by mechanism 2 in Figure 10. This can potentially be impaired by antibiotics

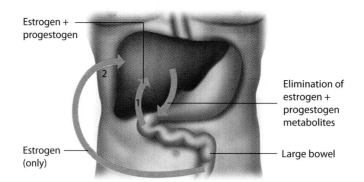

Figure 10
The enterohepatic recirculation of estrogen: (1) 'first pass'—absorption of hormones in the liver; (2) 'second pass'—reabsorption of active estrogen (not progestogen).

that reduce the population of certain gut flora that normally split estrogen metabolites. However, the WHO found that any resulting lowering of EE levels is insufficient for any study to have proven either ovulation or conception as a consequence. It seems this never was a real problem! Presumably, the many previous reports of COC failures because of antibiotics must have been primarily coincidental to missing tablets, which is certainly a common enough factor to coincide. Omissions may additionally occur through vomiting (from the disease or the antibiotic).

WHOMEC and UKMEC therefore advise no restriction on use (WHO 1) of COCs, or more generally CHCs, if there is co-administration of antibiotics that are not enzyme inducers (i.e. other than rifampicin/rifabutin) and therefore no extra precautions are now advised by the British National Formulary as well as the FSRH.

However, they do recommend that women maintain meticulous Pill taking during their illness and are advised about what to do if their antibiotic (or the illness) were to cause vomiting or severe diarrhoea.

Enzyme-inducing drugs
The most clinically important drugs with which this kind of interaction occurs are listed in the following box.

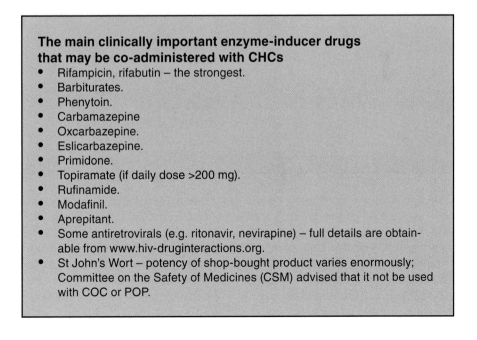

The main clinically important enzyme-inducer drugs that may be co-administered with CHCs
- Rifampicin, rifabutin – the strongest.
- Barbiturates.
- Phenytoin.
- Carbamazepine
- Oxcarbazepine.
- Eslicarbazepine.
- Primidone.
- Topiramate (if daily dose >200 mg).
- Rufinamide.
- Modafinil.
- Aprepitant.
- Some antiretrovirals (e.g. ritonavir, nevirapine) – full details are obtainable from www.hiv-druginteractions.org.
- St John's Wort – potency of shop-bought product varies enormously; Committee on the Safety of Medicines (CSM) advised that it not be used with COC or POP.

Long-term use of enzyme inducers (except rifamycins)

This applies chiefly to epileptic women and women being treated for tuberculosis. This situation is WHO 3, meaning that an alternative method of contraception such as an IUC is preferable – especially for women taking rifampicin or rifabutin, whose effects on the efficacy of CHCs are so strong that long-term users should use another method (WHO 4). Moreover, with the teratogenic anti-epileptic drugs (e.g. rufinamide), pregnancy could be catastrophic.

Much the best options, that should always first be discussed, are the injectable DMPA (with no special advice now needed to shorten the injection interval, see p. 86), an IUD or an LNG-IUS. Implants are not advised (pp. 98–9).

If the woman insists on a COC (*not* the best option):

Only one 50-µg Pill remains on the UK market (see Table 2), and metabolic conversion of the prodrug mestranol to EE is only about 75 per cent efficient. Therefore, Norinyl-1 is almost identical to Norimin. So the FSRH recommends constructing a 50- or 60-µg regimen from two sub-50-µg products (e.g. two tablets daily of Microgynon 30, or e.g. as appropriate, Femodene plus a Femodette® tablet) (see Table 2). As this practice is unlicensed, this is named-patient use, and the guidance on p. 165 should be followed. The woman can be reassured that she is metaphorically 'climbing a down escalator' so as to stay in the right place – her increased liver metabolism meaning that her body should still in reality be receiving a normal low-dose regimen.

Breakthrough bleeding and enzyme-inducer drugs
BTB may occur – indeed, it could be the first clue to a drug interaction. If the long-term user of an enzyme inducer develops persistent BTB, the first step is to exclude another cause (see the D-checklist box on p. 59). Then recommend a 4-day break in the continuous tablet taking. If the problem persists after restarting tablets, a change of method will nearly always be preferable.

The alternative of trying an even higher dose, combining Pills to a total estrogen content of up to 70 µg in an attempt to increase the blood levels of both hormones to above the threshold for bleeding, is not recommended (JG), given uncertainty about the patient's VTE risk (despite the enzyme induction occurring).

Cessation of enzyme inducers after long-term use
It has been shown that 4 or more weeks may elapse before excretory function in the liver reverts to normal. Hence, if any of these drugs has been used for more than 1 month (or at all in the case of rifampicin or rifabutin), there should be a delay of about 4 weeks before returning to a standard low-dose CHC regimen. This period should be increased to 8 weeks after more prolonged use of enzyme inducers. In all cases, there should be no PFI gap between the higher-dose and low-dose packets.

See also useful appendices to the FSRH guidance (URL on p. 54).

Drugs that do *not* pose a clinically important CHC efficacy problem
(despite appearing on past lists, e.g. based only on animal work)
- Griseofulvin.
- Lansoprazole and other proton-pump inhibitors.
- Ethosuximide.
- Valproate.
- Clonazepam.
- Also most newer anti-epileptic drugs not listed here.

Other clinically relevant interacting drugs
Drugs whose own effects may be altered by the COC

- Ciclosporin levels can be raised by COC hormones: The risk of toxic effects means blood levels should be measured.
- Potassium-sparing diuretics: There is a risk of hyperkalaemia with drospirenone, the progestogen in Yasmin (or Daylette, p. 62), so these diuretics should not be used (WHO 4) with those DSP-containing COCs.

- Lamotrigine levels can be lowered by CHCs because of induction by EE of the enzyme glucuronyltransferase which eliminates the anti-epileptic through glucuronidation (see the following box).

Starting a COC in a patient stabilized on a regimen including lamotrigine risks causing an iatrogenic seizure through lowered levels.

- This is WHO 3 – any non–EE-containing contraceptive would definitely be preferable (or a change of anti-epileptic regimen).
- Otherwise, seek her neurologist's advice about a pre-emptive increment in the dose of lamotrigine.
- There is logic in a continuous 365/365 regimen (as earlier) to prevent lamotrigine toxicity, which has been reported as a result of higher blood levels on the rebound in each PFI.
- Exception: If the woman is taking another enzyme inducer as well (because this will already have maximally induced the relevant enzyme) or valproate (which inhibits lamotrigine metabolism).
- There is also no problem in giving lamotrigine to patients already taking a COC because the enzyme is already induced (as earlier), so the dose of anti-epileptic drug may as usual be titrated to the patient's needs.

The lamotrigine dose may need to be lowered when the COC is discontinued, or even during the PFI.

It is all rather complex: hence the ideal is definitely the first bullet here!.

Note: To date (2015), the available evidence supports EE within CHCs as the cause of lowered lamotrigine blood levels, so pending more data any progestogen-only alternative can be offered.

For more information from the FSRH, visit: www.fsrh.org/pdfs/CEUGuidance DrugInteractionsHormonal.pdf.

Counselling and ongoing supervision

Starting the COC

After taking a full personal and family history, with full consideration of possible contraindications on the WHO 1 to 4 scale, as described earlier, each woman deserves individual teaching, backed by the FPA's user-friendly leaflet *Your Guide to the Combined Pill* (as well as by the manufacturer's PIL).

After dealing with the woman's concerns and any questions she may have about risks and benefits – particularly about cancer and circulatory disease – and about 'minor' side effects, the recommended starting routines should be followed as in Table 7 (note the important table footnotes).

Quick-starting

Traditionally, 'medical' methods of contraception such as COCs have been scheduled always to start with or just after the woman's next menstrual period. As discussed on pp. 159–61, this policy is now seen in many cases as having been less than ideal. If the provider can be 'reasonably sure' about the absence of conception risk, it is now accepted, by the WHO, UKMEC and other authorities, as entirely appropriate to advise a woman to start her COC or other medical method on the day she is first seen.

At any time, the user of contraception should be advised about maintaining sexual health. She should be warned, if now or at any future time she knows she is not in a mutually monogamous relationship, to use condoms (ideally supplied on site), in addition to the COC or other 'medical' method. The main take-home messages to be conveyed to a new user are summarized in the following box.

Take-home messages for a new COC taker

- Your FPA leaflet: This is not to be read and thrown away; it is something to keep safely in a drawer somewhere, for ongoing reference.
- The Pill works only if you take it correctly: If you do, each new pack will always start on the same day of the week.
- Even if bleeding, like a 'period', occurs (BTB), carry on Pill taking: Ring for advice if necessary. Nausea is another common early symptom. Both usually settle as your body gets used to the Pill.
- Never be a late restarter of your Pill! Even if your 'period' (withdrawal bleeding) has not stopped yet, never start your next packet late. This is because the PFI is obviously a time when your contraceptive is not being supplied to your ovaries, so they may anyway be beginning to escape from the Pill's actions.
- Lovemaking during the 7 days after any packet is safe only if you do actually go on to the next pack. Otherwise (e.g. if you decide to stop the method), you must start using condoms after the last Pill in the pack.
- For what to do if any Pill(s) are more than 24 hours late (see pp. 45–6).
- Other things that may stop the Pill from working include vomiting and some drugs (always mention that you are on the Pill).
- See a doctor at once if any of the things on p. 65 occur, especially new headaches with strange changes in your eyesight happening beforehand.
- As a one-off, you can shorten one PFI to make sure all your future withdrawal bleeding episodes avoid weekends.
- You can avoid bleeding on holidays and so forth by running packs together. (Discuss this with whomever provides your Pills, if you want to continue missing out 'periods' long term.)
- Good though it is as a contraceptive, the Pill does not give enough protection against *Chlamydia* and other sexually transmitted infections (STIs). Whenever in doubt, especially with a new partner, use a condom as well.
- Finally, always feel free to telephone or come back at any time (maybe to the practice nurse) for any reasons of your own, including any symptoms you would like dealt with.

Note: Very similar advice applies also to users of the other CHCs (i.e. the patch or vaginal ring).

Table 7

Starting routines for combined oral contraceptives

Condition	Start when?	Extra precautions for 7[a] days?
1. Menstruating.	Day 1.	No[b]—if starting with an active tablet.
	Day 2.	No[c]
	Day 3 or later.	Yes (FSRH advises: only from Day 5).
	Sunday start[b].	Yes, unless Sunday = day 1 or 2.
	Any time in cycle ('quick-start').	Yes[d] and if reasonably sure not already conceived or at high conception risk (p. 159).
2. Post-partum status.		
a. No lactation.	Day 21 (low risk of thrombosis by then[e], first ovulations reported day 28+).	No
b. Lactation.	Not normally recommended at all (POP/injectable preferred).	
3. After induced abortion/miscarriage/trophoblastic disease.	Same day—or next day to avoid post-operative vomiting risk. May initiate after first part of any medical abortion. Delay start till Day 21 if was at/beyond 24 weeks' gestation.	No, only needed if COC started >7 days later.
4. After high-dose COC.	Instant switch[f]—or use condoms for 7 days after the PFI.	No
5. After lower- or same-dose COC.	After usual 7-day break, or instantly at choice.	No

56

6. After POP.	First day of period.	No
7. After POP with secondary amenorrhoea, not pregnant.	Any day (Sunday? Has advantages).	No
8. After DMPA, implant, or IUD/IUS (risk of pregnancy excluded).	Any day (see text, usually ideal to overlap the new method with old)	No
9. After IUD/IUS removal, later than D5 in cycle.	Quick-start the COC on day of IUC removal.	Yes, because ovulation still occurs.
10. Other secondary amenorrhoea (risk of pregnancy excluded).	Any day (Sunday?). (Or, quick-starting the COC plus a pregnancy test at 3 weeks is a useful 'ploy', see p. 161)	Yes

Note that FSRH recommendations are slightly less cautious than mine, taking less account of risk of early ovulation in the first cycle.

[a] 9 days for Qlaira (see p. 63).

[b] Everyday (ED) Pill users also start with the first active Pill on day 1. By applying the right sticky strip (out of seven supplied) for that weekday, all future Pills are then labelled with the correct days. A simpler alternative to explain is 'Sunday start', in which the woman delays taking the first active Pill till the first Sunday after her period starts, with condom use sustained through until seven active Pills have been taken. This also ensures that from then onwards there are no bleeds at weekends. (Incidentally, if any COC-user finds these a problem, *having her WTBs only mid-week can be readily ensured by a one-time shortening (by 2–4 days) of her 7-day pill-free interval.*)

[c] Delay into day 2 can sometimes help, to be sure a period is normal, especially after emergency contraception (EC).

[d] Immediate starts – 'Quick-starting' – means starting any day well beyond day 3 (i.e. not waiting as in past practice for that elusive next period); quick-starts are entirely acceptable, provided the prescriber is satisfied there has been no unacceptable conception risk in that cycle (see text here and detailed instructions are at pp. 159–61). EC may sometimes be given first (but **NB special criteria** now (2015) apply if UPA EC is used – see pp. 141–2).

[e] Puerperal risk lasts longer if there are added VTE risk factors, this being WHO 4 till 42 days according to WHOMEC (2015). After severe pregnancy-related hypertension, or the related HELLP syndrome (haemolysis, elevated liver enzymes, low platelets), delay combined hormonal contraceptive (CHC) use until the return of normal blood pressure and biochemistry values. This history in the past is WHO 1.

[f] Perhaps too cautious: but if a 7-day break is taken, there are historical anecdotes of 'rebound ovulation' at time of transfer.

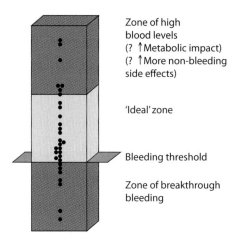

Figure 11
Schematic representation of the marked individual variation in blood levels of both contraceptive steroids.

Second choice of Pill brand

How this relates to the symptom of breakthrough bleeding

Some women react unpredictably, and it is a false expectation that any single Pill will suit all women. Individual variations in motivation and tolerance of minor side effects are well recognized.

However, because of differences in absorption and metabolism, there is also marked variability (threefold, in the area under the curve) in blood levels of the exogenous hormones (Figure 11). This is relevant to the management of irregular bleeding.

Bleeding side effects

Given the 'model' shown in Figure 11 by the variability of blood levels and BTB risk, prescribers should try to identify the lowest dose for each woman that does not cause BTB. This should minimize adverse side effects, both serious and minor, and also reduce measurable metabolic changes. Because COCs all have a powerful contraceptive effect, this approach does not appear to impair effectiveness (far more important is not lengthening the PFI; see earlier). Even if BTB occurs, provided there is ongoing good Pill taking, additional contraception is not needed.

- The objective is that each woman should receive the least long-term metabolic impact that her uterus will allow (i.e. the lowest dose of contraceptive steroids that is only just above her bleeding threshold).
- If BTB does occur and is unacceptable or persists beyond two cycles, a different CHC product may be tried, somewhat empirically, although only after the checks in the so-called 'D-checklist' which follows, p. 59.

The D-checklist for abnormal bleeding in a Pill user

- DISEASE: Consider examining the cervix (it is not unknown for bleeding from an invasive cancer to be wrongly attributed; also a report of BTB should always trigger the thought: *Chlamydia?*).
- DISORDERS of PREGNANCY that cause bleeding (e.g. retained products if the COC was started after a recent termination of pregnancy; or an ectopic [± any pain]). If in doubt, do a pregnancy test.
- DEFAULT: BTB may be triggered 2 or 3 days after a single missed Pills episode and may be persistent thereafter.
- DRUGS, if they are enzyme inducers (see text): Cigarettes are also drugs in this context; BTB has been shown to be statistically more common among smokers.
- Diarrhoea and/or VOMITING: Diarrhoea alone has to be exceptionally severe to impair absorption significantly.
- DISTURBANCES of ABSORPTION: For example, after massive gut resection (rare).
- DURATION of USE too short: BTB after starting on any new formulation may settle, if the pill taker perseveres for 3 months. The opposite may apply during tricycling or other sustained use (see pp. 48–50), namely that the duration of continuous use has been too long for that woman's endometrium to be sustained, in which case a bleeding-triggered break may be taken (p. 50).
- DOSE: After the foregoing have been excluded, it is possible to try
  - A phasic Pill if the woman is receiving monophasic treatment.
  - Increasing first the progestogen then (maybe) the estrogen dose.
  - A different progestogen (evidence – mainly anecdotal – that GSD, DSG and norgestimate [NGM] give better cycle control than LNG Pills); or
- NuvaRing®, which produced less BTB and spotting in the first year of an RCT than Microgynon 30® (Oddsson, 2005; Figure 12).

Modified from Sapire E. *Contraception and Sexuality in Health and Disease.* New York: McGraw-Hill, 1990.

Basically, it is vital first to exclude other causes of BTB, especially D for Disease, before blaming the COC!

Second choice of Pill if there are non-bleeding side effects

- When symptoms occur, it is generally bad practice to give further prescriptions to control them without changing the COC – such as diuretics for weight gain or antidepressants for mood symptoms.
- Aside from trying another CHC (NuvaRing?) or another method, there are two empirical courses of action for problems unrelated to bleeding – to decrease the dose of either hormone, if possible (estrogen can be avoided by trying a POP); or to use a different CHC progestogen.

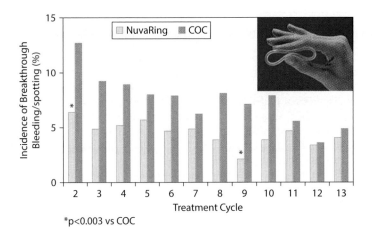

Figure 12
The incidence of breakthrough bleeding + spotting in a randomized controlled trial (n = 1079) comparing NuvaRing with COC (Microgynon 30). (From Oddsson et al. Hum Reprod 2005;20:557–62.)

- Additionally, although the evidence is anecdotal or empirical and there are almost no relevant RCTs, there is a little guidance available for side effects and conditions associated with a relative excess of either sex steroid (see the following boxes).

Which second choice of Pill? Relative estrogen excess

Symptoms
- Nausea.
- Dizziness.
- Leg cramps.
- Cyclical weight gain (fluid-related), 'bloating' – Daylette® is also worth a try here despite its estrogenicity, given the anti-mineralocorticoid activity of drospirenone.
- Vaginal discharge (no infection).
- Some cases of breast enlargement attributed to fluid.
- Some cases of lost libido without depression, theoretically more likely if taking an anti-androgen (but no hard data) – as in Yasmin®, Daylette®, or Dianette® and its generics.

Conditions
- Benign breast disease.
- Fibroids.
- Endometriosis.

For any of these try a progestogen-dominant COC, such as Microgynon 30.

Which second choice of Pill? Relative progestogen excess

Symptoms	Conditions
• Dryness of vagina.	• Acne/seborrhoea.
• Depression/lassitude.	• Hirsutism.
• Depressed mood with or without associated loss of libido.	
• Breast tenderness.	
• Anxiety about weight gain—there is no good evidence that modern COCs cause the weight gain for which they are often blamed.	

Treat with estrogen-dominant COC such as Marvelon or, in moderately severe cases of acne or mild hirsutism, Yasmin or Daylette or co-cyprindiol (see text). Caution is necessary in that their estrogen dominance may correlate with a higher risk of VTE, especially if high BMI (see Table 5, pp. 28–9).

Why choose Yasmin®? Or Daylette®?

Acne, seborrhoea and sometimes hirsutism may be benefited by any of the estrogen-dominant COCs. Yasmin is a monophasic COC containing 3 mg DSP and 30 μg EE. DSP differs from other progestogens in COCs because:

- It is an anti-androgen, so the combination is an alternative to Dianette for the treatment of moderately severe acne and PCOS.
- It has diuretic properties resulting from anti-mineralocorticoid activity.

Yasmin or Daylette are useful options:
- If there is a clear indication for estrogen/anti-androgen therapy, such as moderately severe acne (Marvelon works well for milder cases), including cases associated with PCOS.
- As a useful second choice for empirical control of minor side effects, particularly those associated with fluid retention (e.g. bloatedness and cyclical breast enlargement). Yasmin and Daylette (p. 62) seem to be of value for women with PMS, whether in their normal cycle or also occurring on another COC – continuous use or tricycling being preferable for this indication.
- Last, and definitely least, what about weight? In one study, there was a maintained slight (about 1 per cent) reduction of body mass, but most probably the result of diuresis, hence less total body water compared with controls. Also, if the BMI is already higher than 30, there is a safety issue for any COC – although if Daylette or Yasmin are being given for therapy, the risk/benefit analysis may be different (see pp. 38, 62).

Daylette

Daylette delivers a lower daily dose of ethinylestradiol (20 µg) with drospi-renone 3000 µg. Despite the lower EE dose, its 24/4 regimen with placebos during a 4-day PFI definitely increases efficacy (p. 47). These facts usually make Daylette now preferable on potential safety grounds (see p. 38), for women previously offered Yasmin (JG's view).

What now about co-cyprindiol (marketed *inter alia* as Dianette/Clairette/Acnocin/Cicafem?)

This is another anti-androgenic progestogen plus estrogen combination – co-cyprindiol, with cyproterone acetate (CPA) 2 mg plus EE 35 µg – licensed for the treatment of moderately severe acne and mild hirsutism in women. These are its indications, but practically everything about the COC in this book applies also to Dianette: it is a reliable anovulant, usually giving good cycle control, and has similar rules for missed tablets, interactions, absolute and relative contraindications, and requirements for monitoring.

RCT evidence shows that Yasmin has at least as good effectiveness for the conditions for which Dianette is indicated, and along with Daylette which is so similar these are alternatives that may be used from the outset. Both are estrogen-dominant products requiring careful assessment of VTE risk factors. Given the apparent metabolic 'anti-estrogenicity' of LNG pp. 22–3) the expected relatively increased VTE risk compared with LNG Pills has (2011) been shown for COCs using either DSP or CPA (see p. 24).

Duration of treatment with Dianette® needs to be individualized

In 2013, after the European (EMA) review triggered by VTE concerns about co-cyprindiol in France, the MHRA advised UK clinicians that the estrogen-dominant products using CPA (co-cyprindiol = Dianette + its generic clones) and DSP were higher risk: www.mhra.gov.uk/Safetyinformation/DrugSafetyUpdate/CON287002. It was advised in particular that co-cyprindiol:

- Should be used for moderately severe acne when treatment with topical therapy or systemic antibiotics has failed.
- Should be used only in its licensed indication.
- Should not be used solely for contraception.

In addition,

- An attempt should be made to stop treatment in those with less severe symptoms 3 to 4/12 after they resolve.

(At that point JG's usual practice is to advise Marvelon or its generic, which is often fine for maintenance of improvement; and if not so, usually now switching to Daylette). Advice from the MRHA and BNF continues:

- In all women, co-cyprindiol can be re-started if acne or hirsutism recurs on stopping treatment.
- In women with severe hyperandrogenism co-cyprindiol may be continued until the symptoms are judged unlikely to recur when treatment is stopped. The decision of when to stop treatment may not be easy and should be made on a case-by-case basis using clinical judgement.

How about Qlaira?

This COC contains estradiol valerate (hydrolyzed *in vivo* to natural estradiol [E_2]) and dienogest, a moderately anti-androgenic progestogen. A complicated phasic regimen (four phases plus two lactose placebos; see Table 2) was unavoidable, because of using natural estrogen, which is less potent than EE. With it, there is comparable cycle control to COCs using 20 µg EE. However, users need warning about absent withdrawal bleeding in approximately 20 per cent of cycles.

Maintaining efficacy

There are only 2 days completely hormone-free plus 4 more days of E_2 only, so the manufacturer advises slightly different rules for missed Pills that err very much on the side of caution. Simplified, these are as follows:

If an active tablet is forgotten for more than 12 hours, take it and the next when due, in addition to 9 days of extra precautions. In addition, for late omissions in the pack (days 18 to 24), discard the current wallet and restart a new pack immediately after the omission is recognized – so logically missing out the later days of reduced or absent hormones (see SPC). This advice may change with more experience: even now, a 'missed Pill' could be, as with other COCs, defined as *more than 24 hours late* in my view. EC (specifically LNG EC) should be advised as well (JG's opinion), whenever enough early Pills in a pack have been missed to total more than 9 days in which combined hormones have not been taken and unprotected sexual intercourse (UPSI) also occurred.

Table 7 (pp. 56–7) applies with the one difference that there should be 9 days of added precautions where the right-hand column advises 7 days.

Zoely – a COC with natural estrogen, but monophasic

This consists of 24 white active tablets each containing 2.5 mg nomegestrol acetate and 1.5 mg estradiol (as hemihydrate) with 4 yellow placebo tablets, hence sharing with Qlaira the advantage of a shortened PFI. Its progestogen is highly potent, with similar moderately anti-androgenic activity. Both are effective contraceptives, options (at a price) for any sexually active women; and they usually provide reasonable cycle control with withdrawal bleeding episodes that are short or sometimes absent. Zoely has simpler monophasic packaging than Qlaira, with the same advice for missed pills as for the usual COCs using EE.

Are Qlaira and Zoely safer with respect to thrombosis risk?

Possibly so, because they use the *natural* estrogen E_2, which although still prothrombotic is far less potently so than EE. The total dose of estradiol per 28 days is 52 mg (Qlaira) or 36 mg (Zoely), which is less than in some marketed hormone replacement therapy (HRT) products (56 mg in Kliofem® or Nuvelle®). There is some metabolic evidence of reduced impact on coagulation (e.g. lower blood levels of D-dimer than Pills with 30 µg EE).

So this advantage is *biologically plausible,* but as yet there is *no clinical confirmation* through epidemiology of the hoped-for reduced venous/arterial thrombosis risk.

So when to consider Qlaira or Zoely?

Allowing for their high price and pending more data, Qlaira and Zoely are now the products of choice (JG) *if* a woman will not accept an estrogen-free alternative method and:

- WHO 3 applies in her case for CHCs (e.g. DM with no known 'opathy'; or
- She is late in reproductive life but free of all other known risk factors, from 45 years onward – seeing them in other words as a form of 'contraceptive HRT' up to the age of loss of fertility at the menopause (average age of which is 51 years, maximum age is beyond 55 years; see pp. 161–4).

(However, even better, if acceptable, would be the combination of a lower dose of natural estrogen along with the LNG-IUS.)

Possibly, also, they represent a useful second or third choice of COC for problematic side effects.

Qlaira® is licensed in the United Kingdom – unlike other most other COCs though all have the effect – for treating heavy menstrual bleeding (HMB) without organic pathology. This is based on new data showing 88 per cent reduction compared with baseline in measured menstrual loss (64 per cent versus placebo) after 6 months treatment. So in older women, this is now a good alternative as medical treatment for HMB plus contraception to a LNG-IUS – if the latter is not acceptable.

Stopping COCs

The first menstruation after stopping COCs (for any reason) is often delayed, but not usually for more than about 6 weeks. Secondary amenorrhoea for more than 6 months should always be investigated, whether or not it occurs after stopping COCs – the link will be coincidental and not causal. Whatever the diagnosis, any associated estrogen deficiency should not be allowed to continue long term without treatment.

Listed in the following box are the (only) reasons for discontinuing COCs immediately or soon, and they should be understood by all well-counselled women from their first visit (similar lists are in most PILs, and in the FPA's recommended leaflet *Your Guide to the Combined Pill*). The worst implications of these symptoms are Pill-related thrombotic or embolic catastrophes in the making.

Often there turns out to be another explanation for the symptom, and the COC may be recommenced later. Pending diagnosis, the COC, because of its contained EE, should be stopped, but any progestogen-only method (e.g. Cerazette®) could be started immediately.

Symptoms for which COCs (indeed all CHCs) should be stopped immediately, pending investigation and treatment
- Unusual or severe and very prolonged headache.
- Diagnosis of aura (see above), usually involving loss of part or whole of the field of vision on one side, with or without a migraine following.
- Loss of sight in one eye (unassociated with migraine).
- Disturbance of speech (notably dysphasia in migraine with aura).
- Numbness, severe paraesthesia or weakness on one side of the body (e.g. one arm, side of the tongue); indeed, any symptom suggesting cerebral ischaemia or TIA.
- A severe unexplained fainting attack or severe acute vertigo or ataxia.
- Focal epilepsy.
- Painful swelling in the calf.
- Pain in the chest, especially pleuritic pain.
- Breathlessness or cough with bloodstained sputum.
- Severe abdominal pain.
- Immobilization, for example.
  - After most lower limb fractures; or
  - Major surgery; or
  - Leg surgery.

In all the foregoing circumstances, stop COC, make the diagnosis, and consider anti-thrombotic treatment. If any elective procedure is planned and the Pill is stopped more than 2 weeks ahead (4 weeks is preferable), anti-coagulation is not usually necessary. Contraception can be maintained nowadays by switching to and then later from Cerazette, or another brand of desogestrel POP, which is believed to have negligible prothrombotic effects.

Other reasons for speedy discontinuation:
- Acute jaundice.
- BP higher than 160/95 mm Hg on repeated measurement (p. 39).
- Severe skin rash (erythema multiforme).
- Detection of a significant new risk factor or interacting disease (e.g. onset of severe SLE, first diagnosis of breast cancer).

Pill follow-up: what is important?

Aside from the management of established risk factors or diseases already present, or that may suddenly or more gradually appear, and of new minor side effects (both dealt with earlier), follow-up primarily entails two items of monitoring:

- Blood pressure; and
- Headaches, especially migraine.

Blood pressure

Monitoring of BP is vital. It should be recorded before COCs are started and checked after 3 months (1 month in a high-risk case) and subsequently at intervals of, initially, 6 months. COCs should always be stopped altogether if BP increase is entirely COC related and exceeds 160/95 mm Hg on repeated measurements (p. 39). A more moderate increase still suggests the possibility of an increased risk of arterial disease, especially in the presence of any other arterial risk factors (see Table 6).

However, if a low-risk COC taker remains normotensive, with no rise between successive measurements during (in my view) the first 6–9 months (UKMEC proposes this as soon as after the 3-month visit), taking the BP of COC users annually should now be the norm – in women developing no risk factors. This is good practice so long as it is made abundantly clear that they may return sooner for advice, as and when they may wish – a truly 'open-house' policy.

Headaches

Not to ask about a COC taker's headaches at any regular or requested Pill follow-up visit would be a serious omission (see pp. 39–42 for the crucial importance of identifying migraine with aura and how to do it).

Screening

Note what is not included earlier in the follow-up requirements: neither breast and bimanual pelvic examinations nor monitoring blood tests have any relevance to Pill follow-up. Routine bimanual pelvic examinations in asymptomatic COC takers are particularly uncalled for, because the disorders causing detectable pelvic masses or tenderness are all actually less frequent in COC takers than in others, as listed on p. 16.

Even taking cervical smears is for screening and not primarily a COC-associated exercise. After the age of 25 years, cervical screening should simply be performed regularly, as guidelines recommend for all sexually active women.

Congenital abnormalities and fertility issues

Any possible effect of COCs on congenital abnormalities is difficult to establish because it is so difficult to prove a negative; moreover, 2 per cent of all full-term fetuses have a significant malformation.

- Even with exposure during organogenesis, meta-analyses of the major studies fail to show an increased risk. If present, it must be very small.
- When COCs are used before the conception cycle, the conclusions of a WHO scientific group have not since been challenged – namely, that there is no good evidence for any adverse effects on the fetus of COCs. It can do no harm if a woman stops COCs and switches to barriers for 2 or more months before conception, but there is no objective evidence that it is worth the effort. Certainly, any woman who finds herself pregnant immediately after stopping COCs should be strongly reassured.

What about 'taking breaks' to optimize fertility?

Concerns about its reversibility have dogged the COC since its first marketing. Fertile ovulation can be minimally delayed on cessation, for a matter of days or up to 4 weeks – a much shorter time than following injectable use (see later). Yet, just as for the latter method, there is no evidence that COCs can cause permanent loss of fertility. Indeed, a large study (*Hum Reprod* 2002;17:2754–61) showed that use of the COC for more than 5 years before the 8497 planned conceptions was associated with a *decreased* risk of delay in conceiving.

There is even some evidence of harm from an intake break of 4 or more weeks, namely increased VTE risk when re-starting use (p. 26).

If a woman still feels more comfortable to take a routine break from the COC, we should always help her to find a satisfactory contraceptive alternative. However, she should understand there is no known benefit from taking short elective breaks of 6 months or so every few years, as was admittedly once recommended.

In one study, one fourth of young women who took breaks as noted earlier had unwanted conceptions. Relevantly, another finding of the *Human Reproduction* report quoted earlier was that one third of the whole population admitted their pregnancy was not truly planned – and this was a population surveyed in antenatal clinics, and thus could not include those who had pregnancies terminated.

Summary
- The first visit for prescription of COCs is by far the most important, and should never be rushed. A second visit in the first week, to the same or maybe a different provider in the surgery, provides a valuable opportunity for questions.
- The LARCs, long-term and 'forgettable' contraceptive options, should always be included in the discussion, despite the woman's presenting request for what she happens to know about (most probably the Pill).
- If the Pill remains her choice, along with discussing the risks and benefits, and fully assessing her medical and family history – all at her level of understanding – there is much ground to cover (see the 'Take-home messages' list earlier). Often it is useful to share this between the doctor and practice or clinic nurse.
- Thereafter, there are really only three key components to COC monitoring during follow-up, which is primarily annual (p. 66) but with 'open house' access upon request:
  - BP.
  - Headaches.
  - Identification and management of any new risk factors/diseases/side effects.

No matter how carefully those with contraindications are excluded, a few women will experience adverse effects. Repeated presentation with multiple side effects sometimes suggests the offer of a different method rather than a different Pill – or, that a psychosexual problem needs to be faced.

For more, including most references for this chapter, visit: www. fsrh.org/pdfs/CEUGuidanceCombinedHormonalContraception.pdf.

TRANSDERMAL COMBINED HORMONAL CONTRACEPTION: EVRA®

Evra® is a transdermal patch delivering EE with norelgestromin, the active metabolite of NGM. The daily skin dose of 33.9 µg EE with 203 µg norelgestromin is intended to produce blood levels in the reference range of those after a tablet of Cilest but without either the diurnal fluctuations or the oral peak dose given to the liver.

Pending more data, all the absolute and relative contraindications and indeed most of the foregoing practical management advice in Chapters 5 and 6 about the COC apply to this CHC, with obvious minor adjustments. It can be seen as a bit like 'Cilest through the skin'.

However, in the United States, the Food and Drug Administration (FDA) requires a warning in the Evra SPC, initially based on its pharmacokinetics, that patch users are exposed to about 60 per cent more total estrogen;

moreover, a majority of case-control studies showed an increased risk of VTE, compared with oral COCs with 30 to 35 µg estrogen. In other studies, Evra also produced relatively more estrogen-associated side effects such as breast tenderness and nausea. The FDA concluded (2008) that 'Ortho Evra is a safe and effective method of contraception when used according to the labelling' but advises added caution for women with VTE risk factors.

In studies, the patch had excellent adhesion even in hot climates and when bathing or showering; the incidence of detachment of patches was 1.8 per cent (complete) and 2.9 per cent (partial). About 2 per cent of women had local skin reactions that led to discontinuation. In the pooled analysis of three pivotal studies (*Fertil Steril* 2002;[2 suppl 2]), the Pearl index for consistent users of Evra was similar to that for oral Pills – and less than 1 per 100 woman-years.

Interestingly, in the clinical trials, one third of the few failures occurred in the 3 per cent of women weighing more than 90 kg. In my view, this apparently reduced effectiveness contraindicates (WHO 4) Evra for such women, when added to the VTE risk from the BMI they are likely to have weighing 90 kg, anyway. They are far from ideal users of this estrogen-dominant product.

Maintenance of efficacy of Evra®

- Avoid use at all if body weight >90 kg, indeed in all cases with a risk factor for VTE – on safety as well as efficacy grounds.
- Warn the user that the contraceptive is in the glue of the patch, so a dry patch that has fallen off should not be re-used!
- Each patch is worn for 7 days, for 3 consecutive weeks, followed by a patch-free week. This regimen was shown to aid compliance, particularly in young women. Before age 20, 'perfect use' was reported in 68 per cent of COC cycles, but in 88 per cent of patch cycles. Clinically, the patch, along with NuvaRing described later, is therefore an alternative to offer to those who, refusing a LARC, find it difficult to remember a daily Pill. Usefully, there is a 2-day margin for error for late patch change. Setting up a weekly mobile text reminder 'Today is your new patch day' can also help.
- As with the COC, it is essential never to lengthen the contraception-free (patch-free) interval.
- If this interval exceeds 8 days for any reason (either through late application or through the first new patch detaching and this being identified late), advise extra precautions for the duration of the first freshly applied patch (i.e. for 7 days), usually LNG EC (see pp. 141–2, 147), should be considered if there has been sexual exposure during the preceding patch-free time, and that *exceeded 9 days*.
- Absorption problems through vomiting/diarrhoea have no effect on this method's efficacy, but:
- During short-term enzyme-inducer therapy, and for 28 days after this ends, additional contraception (e.g. with condoms) is advised, plus elimination of any patch-free intervals during this time. For long-term therapy, advise another method: use of two patches at a time is not advised (UKMEC).

TRANSVAGINAL COMBINED HORMONAL CONTRACEPTION: NUVARING

NuvaRing is a combined vaginal ring depicted in Figure 12 (p. 60) that releases etonogestrel (3-ketodesogestrel) 120 µg and EE 15 µg/day, thus equating to some degree with 'vaginal Mercilon'. It is normally retained for 3 weeks and then removed for withdrawal bleeding during the fourth week. There is an option to remove it for up to 3 hours during sex, with extra precautions advised only if it is absent for longer.

It should not be used by women with significant vaginal prolapse. Otherwise, expulsion is uncommon, occurring usually in parous women, in only 2.3 per cent in the first 13 cycles of a trial, of which 1.7 per cent occurred in the first 3 cycles (N = 3333). The instruction to users is just to wash it and reinsert; this rarely means that women must change method.

Pending more dedicated information, all the absolute and relative contraindications, and most of the foregoing practical management advice about the COC, apply also to this CHC. It appears to have a side effect profile very like that of Mercilon itself.

In studies, it proved very popular, with maintained sexual satisfaction, excellent cycle control (see Figure 12, p. 60) and a failure rate comparable to that of oral COCs.

It was also found (*Contraception* 2006;73:488–92) that 'baseline discomfort with genital touching' was not a problem.

Maintenance of efficacy of NuvaRing
- Expulsions occurred primarily during the emptying of bowels or bladder and therefore were readily recognized.
- As with the COC, it remains essential never to lengthen the contraception-free (ring-free) interval. If for any reason this exceeds 8 days, advise extra precautions for 7 days. As for Evra, EC – usually LNG EC (see p. 141–2, 147) – should be considered if there has been sexual exposure during any ring-free time that exceeds 9 days.
- Advise as routine a day 28 ring-insertion reminder by mobile phone!
- Also, because the ring when *in situ* is imperceptible to the user, the suggestion to make it part of foreplay to check that it is there before sex may prevent some failures.
- Absorption problems and vomiting or diarrhoea have no detectable effect on this method's efficacy.
- During short-term enzyme-inducer therapy and afterward for 28 days, additional contraception is advised, in addition to elimination of any ring-free intervals. For long-term therapy, advise another method.

Comparison between ring and patch – the ring seems to have the edge	
Ring	**Patch**
EE blood levels—area under the curve lower: 3.4 × that in ring users cpd with patch; 2.1 × cpd with COC.	EE blood levels higher by 60 per cent compared with 35 µg norgestimate COC
Less nausea and breast tenderness than patch or an EE-dominant COC, so ring better choice if high BMI.	Confirms patch is more estrogenic. Method best avoided if VTE risk. Also risk of failure in obesity (see text).
Expulsions occur (see text; continuation usually possible).	Patches can fall off.
Vaginal symptoms reported more with ring; not thrush or STIs.	Skin reactions can cause discontinuation.
(? Lowered threshold to report?).	
In United States, RCT recruiting from COC users; 71 per cent ring users vs. 27 per cent patch users wished to go on using, rather than return to COC (Creinin *et al. Obstet Gynecol* 2008).	
Better cycle control than 30 µg LNG-COC (see Fig. 12, p. 60).	

However these methods share some advantages:

- Some women find them easier to remember than a daily COC.
- Their effectiveness cannot be reduced by vomiting.
- There is an absorption advantage, if there is concern about reduced COC absorption in the upper small bowel such as after massive gut resection or in severe Crohn's disease (p. 37).

Progestogen-only pill

There are four varieties of POP available (Table 8): three are of the old type of products that variably inhibit ovulation, whereas the fourth, Cerazette®, is a primarily anovulant product. Several other brand names of the latter are now marketed, hence we shall now routinely refer to this as the DSG POP. Unless otherwise stated, the abbreviation POP will refer to the three old-type POPs. The excellent FSRH Guidance on POPs is available at www.fsrh.org/pdfs/CEUGuidanceProgestogenOnlyPills.pdf where, as usual, references to studies mentioned here can be found.

MECHANISM OF ACTION AND MAINTENANCE OF EFFECTIVENESS

The mechanism of action is complex because of variable interactions between the administered progestogen and the endogenous activity of the woman's ovary. Outside of lactation (when their effectiveness is hugely enhanced; see later), fertile ovulation is prevented in 50 to 60 per cent of cycles. In the remainder, there is reliance mainly on progestogenic interference with mucus penetrability. This 'barrier' effect is readily lost, so that each old-type POP tablet must be taken within 3 hours of the same regular time.

If POPs are indeed taken each day within that time span of 27 hours, without breaks and regardless of bleeding patterns, they are in practice as effective (or as ineffective, in 'typical use; see Table 1!) as COCs – especially for women 35 years old and older.

Effectiveness

In the United Kingdom, the Oxford/Family Planning Association study reported a failure rate for old-type POPs of 3.1 per 100 woman-years between the ages 25 and 29 years, but this improved to 1.0 at 35 to 39 years of age and was as low as 0.3 for women older than 40 years of age. Realistically, most users are probably not as meticulous as those married middle-class women.

Table 8
Available POPs

Product	Active constituent	Course of treatment
Noriday®	350 µg norethisterone	28 tablets
Micronor®	350 µg norethisterone	28 tablets
Norgeston®	30 µg levonorgestrel	35 tablets
DSG POPs* (many brands)	75 µg desogestrel	28 tablets

*In United Kingdom, branded as Aizea®, Cerazette®, Cerelle®, Desomono®, Desorex®, Nacrez®, Zelleta®.

The DSG POP is very different because it blocks ovulation in 97 per cent of cycles and had a failure rate in the pre-marketing study of only 0.17 per 100 woman-years (in consistent users even without breastfeeding).

With regard to effect of body mass (not BMI), studies are suggestive, but not conclusive, that the failure rate of old-type POPs may be higher with increasing weight, as was well established in early studies of progestogen rings and some implants. Pending more data, a logical policy now is to make the DSG POP one's first choice for women weighing more than 70 kg (irrespective of height), especially if they are young. This is preferable to taking two POPs, although that is still an off-licence option.

However, because of reduced fertility, there can be little doubt that one old-type POP daily will be adequately effective in older overweight women, in women older than 45 years, or during established breastfeeding.

Missed pills

Loss of full contraceptive activity through missed Pills or vomiting (without successful replacement of the vomited tablet) is believed to start within as little as 3 hours, or 12 hours for the DSG POP. After restarting, for how long should extra precautions then be advised? Two days for all POPs is 'traditional' and still (2015) advised by the FSRH. The SPCs all advise 7 days. The uncertainty here is discussed in an important Footnote (JG) on p. 82.

Clinically, after missing a POP for more than 3 hours (or after more than 12 hours for the DSG POP; see later) the woman should:
- Take that day's Pill immediately and the next one on time.
- Use added precautions for the next 2 days (FSRH) or 7 days (advised in all SPCs). See p. 82.

Additionally, with old-type POPs, if there has already been intercourse without added protection between the time of first potential loss of the mucus effect through to its restoration by 48 hours, it is appropriate to:
- Advise immediate emergency contraception (EC), usually with levonorgestrel (see pp. 141–2, 147, 149), with the next old-type POP taken on time.

What EC action is needed during full lactation in women taking ordinary POPs, or for DSG POP users (who rely less on the mucus effect and have at least 12 hours of 'leeway' anyway)?

Here there is established anovulation (moreover, without any of the COCs' Pill-free intervals, with their contraception-weakening effect). So although the first two bullets in the foregoing box would apply, EC would be needed less often than implied in the box (i.e. not in the majority of cases).

LACTATION

According to the lactational amenorrhoea method (LAM – see Figure 20), even without the POP, there is only about a 2 per cent conception risk if all three LAM criteria continue to apply.

LAM criteria:
- Amenorrhoea, because the lochia ceased.
- Full lactation – the baby's nutrition is effectively all from its mother.
- Baby not yet 6 months old.

This is why, when women are taking any POP (old-type or DSG POP) during full lactation, EC is very rarely indicated for missed POPs. However, because breastfeeding varies in its intensity, if an old-type POP tablet is 3 hours late, it is still usual to advise additional precautions during the next 2 tablet-taking days.

What dose to the baby?

During lactation, with all POPs (including the DSG POP), the dose to the infant is believed to be harmless, but this aspect must always be discussed. The least amount of administered progestogen enters the breast milk if the highly protein-bound LNG POP (Norgeston®) is used. The quantity has been calculated to be the equivalent of one POP in 2 years – considerably less than the progesterone of cow's milk origin found in formula feedings.

If EC is required (exceptionally [see earlier], perhaps because of multiple Pill omissions) by a breastfeeding mother, once again very little LNG reaches the breast milk. She may wish to express and discard her breast milk for 8 to 12 hours; the dose reaching her baby will become negligible thereafter.

Weaning

Beware – unwanted conceptions are common when lactating POP users have not been adequately warned that their margin for error in POP taking will diminish at weaning. This is one reason for using the DSG POP, to maintain efficacy as lactational infertility wanes. Users of other POPs should be given a supply of a 'stronger' method, such as the COC or the DSG POP, in good time, along with clear instructions to start it when breast milk stops being their baby's main nutrition, or no later than the first bleeding.

Drug interactions

A reminder: broad-spectrum antibiotics do not interfere with the effectiveness of any hormonal method.

- Enzyme inducers: Another contraceptive method is advised during use of liver enzyme inducers such as rifampicin or carbamazepine and continuing after stopping for at least 4 weeks (see earlier, regarding COCs, pp. 51–3). Long-term treatment with enzyme inducers is classified as WHO 3 and the FSRH advises an injectable or IUC. However, if a suitable alternative contraceptive is not identified and the couple does not wish to use condoms indefinitely, increasing the dose is an option (my view [JG], not UKMEC) – usually to two DSG POPs daily, after assessing all relevant factors including lactation and the woman's body weight, age and likely fertility. This is unlicensed use (p. 165).

- Bosentan: This endothelin antagonist is an enzyme-inducing drug that would never be relevant for any CHC because it is used to treat pulmonary hypertension (which is WHO 4 for CHCs). However, the DSG POP could be an option for a young woman with this serious condition – again with two tablets (JG, not UKMEC) taken daily to compensate for the enzyme induction. Double-dosing use is always unlicensed.

Note: Better than the foregoing unlicensed double dosing, especially given that pregnancy can be lethal in pulmonary hypertension, would be the use of DMPA or an IUD or IUS, which is always a preferred contraceptive where there is enzyme induction (p. 86).

ADVANTAGES

In terms of health, because POPs are EE free, these are exceptionally safe products. There are negligible changes to most metabolic variables. There is no proven causative link with any of the following:

- Any tumour (there was a non-significant increase in breast cancer risk in the 1996 Collaborative Group Study (p. 17), which has not been confirmed).
- Venous or arterial disease.
- Osteopenia, weight gain, depression or headache.

INDICATIONS

See the following box for indications. Some of them are WHO 2 and not WHO 1, but that always means 'broadly usable', hence an indication if a Pill method is wanted and a COC would be WHO 3 or WHO 4:

Indications for POP or DSG POP use
- Woman's choice: the DSG POP should no longer now be seen as a 'second-choice' method, for use only when a COC is contraindicated or unacceptable.
- Lactation, where the combination even with ordinary POPs is extra effective – indeed as good as the COC would be in non-breastfeeders.
- Side effects with, or recognized contraindications to, the combined Pill, in particular where estrogen related. Because EE-free products do not appear to affect blood-clotting mechanisms significantly, POPs may be used (WHO 2) by women with a definite past history of VTE and a whole range of disorders predisposing to both arterial and venous disease (WHO 2). Good counselling and record keeping are essential.
- Major or leg surgery or over the time of treatments for varicose veins – when COCs are often contraindicated on VTE grounds (WHO 2).
- Sickle cell disease, severe structural heart disease or pulmonary hypertension (DSG is the preferred progestogen on efficacy grounds).
- Smokers older than 35 years, onward until the menopause.
- Hypertension, whether COC related or not, controlled on treatment.
- Migraine, including varieties with aura (WHO 2: the woman may well continue to suffer migraines, but the fear of an EE-promoted thrombotic stroke is eliminated). The DSG POP is preferred, to obtain optimum stability of endogenous hormones whose fluctuation may cause attacks.
- Diabetes mellitus – but caution WHO 3 if there is significant DM with tissue damage (see later).
- Obesity – but then usually prescribing the DSG POP (see text).

Old-type POPs are still good during lactation and for the older woman, given diminished fertility; but for the young, highly fertile woman, the DSG POP is now the POP of choice.

RISKS AND DISADVANTAGES

Side effects

The main side effect of POPs and the DSG POP is irregular bleeding, about which all prospective users should be clearly warned.

The irregularity can include oligo-amenorrhoea. This occurs more commonly with the DSG POP than with other POPs. However, reassuringly, it appears that with all POPs, the DSG POP and Nexplanon®, follicle-stimulating hormone (FSH) is not completely suppressed even during the amenorrhoea, which is mainly caused by luteinizing hormone (LH) suppression. There is therefore enough follicular activity at the ovary to maintain adequate mid-follicular phase estrogen levels. Pending more data, this means that there is not the concern about bone density reduction that exists for DMPA (see later).

For management of side effects during follow-up, see later.

CONTRAINDICATIONS

Absolute contraindications (WHO 4) for POP and DSG POP use
- Any serious adverse effect of CHCs not certainly related solely to the estrogen (e.g. liver adenoma or cancer, although FSRH says UKMEC 3).
- Recent breast cancer not yet clearly in remission (see later).
- Hypersensitivity to any component.
- Current pregnancy.
- WHO 3 conditions for POP and DSG POP use.
- Current ischaemic heart disease, severe arterial diseases including stroke.
- Sex steroid–dependent cancer, including breast cancer, when in complete remission (UKMEC categorises it WHO 4 until 5 years, then 3). Agreement of the relevant hospital consultant should be obtained and the woman's autonomy respected: record that she understands it is unknown whether progestogen may alter the recurrence risk (either way).
- Severe liver disease (acute viral hepatitis, decompensated cirrhosis).
- Acute porphyria, if there is a history of an actual attack triggered by hormones (my view, because progestogens as well as estrogens are believed capable of precipitating these attacks, and 1 per cent of the attacks are fatal). Otherwise, a history of acute porphyria is WHO 2 for all POPs.
- Previous treatment for ectopic pregnancy in a nulliparous woman; however, this can be an indication for the DSG POP! Despite a 1 in 10 risk that 'breakthrough' pregnancies will be ectopic, the overall risk of recurrent ectopic pregnancy is reduced among old-type POP users, which is why the condition is actually classified as UKMEC 1. However, in my view, it would be much better here to offer the COC, DMPA, the DSG POP, or Nexplanon than a POP because the risk can be reduced still further by methods that regularly block fertilization – to better preserve the precious remaining fallopian tube.
- Undiagnosed genital tract bleeding until cause established.
- Enzyme inducers: although in my view two POPs can be taken, off-licence (see earlier), another method such as an injectable, IUD or LNG-IUS would again be preferable.

There remain some conditions where the POP method is generally WHO 2. These may even be *indications* when other effective alternatives are rejected:

COUNSELLING AND ONGOING SUPERVISION

The starting routines are summarized in Table 9. Crucial aspects of counselling are as follows:

- Clarity for earlier COC users that they should not take a 7-day break after 21 days! Every year because of the lack of this information, there occur what can only be termed 'iatrogenic' conceptions.
- Passing on the tip to dedicate one mobile phone alarm or text message to 'POP- taking time'.

Frequent or prolonged menstrual bleeding

This is the main nuisance side effect. With advance warning, it may be tolerated. Improvement appears more likely with the DSG POP, based on the randomized controlled trial comparing it with an LNG POP. By 1 year, around half of ongoing DSG POP users reported amenorrhoea (which with counselling can be accepted as an advantage) or infrequent bleeding (one or two bleeding episodes per 90 days).

In this pre-market study, however, the improved bleeding pattern was evident only when users persevered beyond 6 months, and no treatment for prolonged or heavy bleeding is reliably effective. Having excluded a coincidental cause (based on the D-checklist on p. 59), taking two tablets daily (or

Table 9

Starting routines for POPs

Condition before start	Start when?	Extra precautions?
Menstruation	Day 1 of period	No
	Days 2–5	No
	Any time in cycle ('quick-start')	2 days or 7 days[a]
Post-partum		
No lactation	Usually day 21 (can be earlier)	No
Lactation	Day 21 – maybe later if 100 per cent lactation (UKMEC recommends) delay till 6 weeks)	No
After induced abortion/ miscarriage	Same day[b]	No
After COCs	Instant switch	No
Amenorrhoea (e.g. post-partum)	Any time[c]	2 days or 7 days[a]

[a]Can start any day in selected cases if the prescriber is satisfied there has been negligible conception risk up to the starting day. NB: 7 days of extra precautions are advised in the SPC (and must be even more effective if complied with). The evidence base for 2 days is weak, so JG now prefers 7 days (p. 82). NB if EC using UPA is given, first, see pp. 141–2.
[b]Ovulation has been shown on Day 8 after 1st trimester abortion. FSRH guidance (2015) advises, also, that 'hormonal contraceptives can be initiated after the *first* part of a medical abortion'.
[c]Even if recent UPSI, with pregnancy test negative, and a further pregnancy test arranged 3 weeks later. POPs are not thought to be teratogenic (see pp. 159–61).

one tablet twice daily) can be successful, anecdotally, often enough to be worth a trial (JG and see p. 165). However a change of method is more usual.

Amenorrhoea

Except during full lactation, prolonged spells of amenorrhoea occur most often in older women. Once pregnancy has been excluded, the amenorrhoea must be the result of anovulation, and so it signifies very high efficacy – as well as convenience for many women, without evidence of harm.

Non-bleeding side effects

These side effects are rare with POPs, apart from the following complaints:

- Breast tenderness, although common, is usually transient; if it recurs, it can sometimes be overcome by changing to the DSG POP.

- Functional cysts or luteinized unruptured follicles are also not uncommon; however, most are symptomless, and pelvic pain on one or the other side is relatively unusual.

Clinically, if functional cysts among POP users do become symptomatic, they can lead to problems in the differential diagnosis of ectopic pregnancy (pain, menstrual disturbance and a tender adnexal mass present in both conditions).

Monitoring

The BP of all POP takers is checked initially, but thereafter if not raised it does not need to be taken more often than for other women. POP takers need no regular visits – just the usual 'open-house' policy, the freedom to discuss any problems on request. If the BP was raised during COC use, it usually reverts to normal on POPs. If it does not, indeed, the woman most probably has essential hypertension.

Return of fertility after discontinuing POPs, including the DSG POP

This is rapid: indeed clinically, from the user's point of view, fertility after stopping must be assumed to be immediate.

Menopause

Establishing ovarian failure at the menopause is less important than with CHCs because all the POPs are safe enough products to continue using well into the sixth decade, usually in fact to beyond age 55 years, when loss of fertility is almost invariable, as discussed later (pp. 162–3). First switching to any POP from any other hormonal method, and then continuing until that age, can be a reassuring way to manage that often difficult transition out of the reproductive years.

In women taking any type of POP, the FSRH advises that, if amenorrhoea and vasomotor symptoms appear after the age of 50 years, a high blood FSH measurement (>30 IU/L) suggests ovarian failure. This may then be confirmed by following Plan C on page 164.

However, if the FSH is found to be low, this suggests (despite the amenorrhoea) continuing ovarian function. If the POP is not simply continued to that age of more than 55 years when ovarian function is usually negligible, another effective contraceptive needs to be used until loss of fertility is finally established (pp. 161–4).

MORE ABOUT THE DSG POP

Mechanism of action and maintenance of effectiveness

This product contains 75 µg desogestrel and to some extent 'rewrites the textbooks' about POPs – mainly because it blocks ovulation in 97 per cent of cycles and had a failure rate in the pre-marketing study of only 0.17 per 100 woman-years (and that without also breastfeeding). This makes it somewhat like 'Nexplanon by mouth'.

Following a reassuring European study, in which DSG POP tablets were deliberately taken late, 12 hours of 'leeway' in Pill taking have been approved before extra precautions are advised – these then being either for 2 days (FSRH advice), based on the sperm-blocking effect of progestogens on cervical mucus, the concept that all POPs are a bit like 'barrier contraceptives that you swallow'; or for 7 days as the manufacturer's SPC still recommends (see p. 82). This has led in recent years to a surge in the popularity of the DSG POP among young and highly fertile users for whom we would previously not even have suggested a POP.

Otherwise, the DSG POP shares the medical safety and rapid reversibility – but also, unfortunately, the tendency to irregular bleeding side effects and functional ovarian cyst formation – of the old-type POPs.

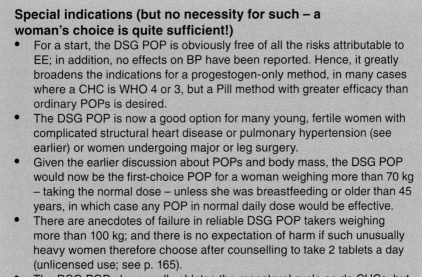

Special indications (but no necessity for such – a woman's choice is quite sufficient!)

- For a start, the DSG POP is obviously free of all the risks attributable to EE; in addition, no effects on BP have been reported. Hence, it greatly broadens the indications for a progestogen-only method, in many cases where a CHC is WHO 4 or 3, but a Pill method with greater efficacy than ordinary POPs is desired.
- The DSG POP is now a good option for many young, fertile women with complicated structural heart disease or pulmonary hypertension (see earlier) or women undergoing major or leg surgery.
- Given the earlier discussion about POPs and body mass, the DSG POP would now be the first-choice POP for a woman weighing more than 70 kg – taking the normal dose – unless she was breastfeeding or older than 45 years, in which case any POP in normal daily dose would be effective.
- There are anecdotes of failure in reliable DSG POP takers weighing more than 100 kg; and there is no expectation of harm if such unusually heavy women therefore choose after counselling to take 2 tablets a day (unlicensed use; see p. 165).
- The DSG POP also usually ablates the menstrual cycle as do CHCs, but without using EE. So it has potentially beneficial effects and can be tried (but not always successfully – no promises possible) in a range of disorders, including: past history of ectopic pregnancy (discussed earlier); dysmenorrhoea; mittelschmerz; and premenstrual syndrome.

Starting routines

See Table 9 (i.e. as other POPs).

Problems and disadvantages

As with all progestogen-only methods, irregular bleeding remains a very real problem. Indeed, this is the one area showing no great advantage in the pre-marketing comparative study with LNG 30-µg POP users. The dropout rate for changes in bleeding pattern showed no difference, but among those women who persevered, there was a useful trend for the more annoying frequent and prolonged bleeding experiences to lessen with continued use.

Despite this higher incidence of (more acceptable) oligo-amenorrhoea than with existing POPs, the DSG POP (like other POPs and Nexplanon) appears to continue to provide adequate follicular phase levels of estradiol for bone health (p. 94).

Contraindications

These contraindications, whether WHO 4, 3 or 2, are very similar to those for the old-type POPs listed earlier. The main difference is that the DSG POP is more effective, making it positively suitable for some with a past history of ectopic pregnancy.

> **In summary:**
> The DSG POP has now become a first-line hormonal contraceptive for many women. However, there is no strong indication for its use in full lactation or for older women who are older than 45 years. One cannot expect to improve on 100 per cent contraception, which these two states do (almost) provide, even when combined with an old-type POP.

FOOTNOTE: ANTICIPATED TIME TO ESTABLISH RELIABLE CONTRACEPTION AFTER STARTING OR RE-STARTING THE DSG POP, OR OTHER POPs

For how long should extra precautions be advised? Two days for all POPs is 'traditional' and still (2015) advised by the FSRH. Yet the evidence that 2 days is enough time, to create a sperm-impermeable mucus barrier in all or nearly all women, is not confirmed in all studies. Moreover accepted practice is to advise added precautions for 7 days when starting, at any time in the cycle, ovulation-blocking contraceptives such as the COC (pp. 44–6). All POPs have that potential, strongest in the DSG POP, so in my view (JG), why not play safer and recommend 7 days for them also? That is also, usefully, congruent with the SPCs for all marketed POPs.

Injectables

BACKGROUND

In the United Kingdom, the only injectable currently licensed for long-term use is DMPA – given as Depo-Provera®, 150 mg intramuscularly or Sayana® Press, 104 mg subcutaneously. Since 2014 it has become a normal option to give these every 13 weeks (this is the licensed interval subcutaneously, but is unlicensed at present for intramuscular DMPA).

For this and further information on injectables and all key references, see the FSRH Guidance, available at www.fsrh.org/pdfs/CEUGuidanceProgestogenOnlyInjectables.pdf.

Despite early campaigns against its use, this method has been repeatedly endorsed by the expert committees of prestigious bodies, such as the International Planned Parenthood Federation (IPPF) and WHO. There is concern about a few issues such as osteoporosis, but DMPA is without doubt (even) safer than combined hormonal contraceptives (CHCs).

DMPA is not associated with any risk of ovarian or endometrial cancer and, indeed, like CHCs, is likely to offer some protection. Some studies have not ruled out a weak causative link with breast cancer from current use, but returning with time after stopping toward normal risk. There is a weak association between cervical cancer and use of DMPA for 5 years or longer, but this could be the result of confounding factors such as number of sexual partners and HPV exposure. Reassuringly, the overall risk of cancer seems, from WHO studies, to be reduced by DMPA use.

A number of 'medical' myths or half-truths about this method persist and will be dealt with below. For example:

- That it causes infertility
- That hypo-estrogenism and osteopenia are very common
- That, in particular, it should not be used in young teenagers soon after the menarche, because it will seriously impair either pituitary/ovarian function or their achieving of peak bone density.

ADMINISTRATION

Intramuscular route

DMPA 150 mg is given every 12 or 13 weeks (sometimes less; see later), and norethisterone enantate or NET-EN (Noristerat®) 200 mg is given every 8 weeks. After the pre-loaded syringe for the former is well shaken and the ampoule for the latter, which is oily, is pre-warmed, each is given by deep intramuscular injection in the first 5 days of the menstrual cycle. First injections (of the subcutaneous injection [see the next section] as well) may also be given in special cases (see p. 160) beyond day 5, with 7 days of added precautions, if it is sufficiently certain that a conception risk has not been taken (p. 158). The injection sites, in the United Kingdom, are usually in the upper outer quadrant of either buttock, although the upper outer thigh and deltoid are also acceptable sites; these sites should not be massaged.

Noristerat is not licensed for long-term contraception, although it can be so used off-licence (p. 165). It is not considered further here.

Subcutaneous route

DMPA 104 mg is injected under the skin of the abdominal wall or upper thigh. This is Sayana Press (Depo-subQ Provera 104® in the United States), supplied in a small bubble of clear plastic (Figure 13) pre-filled with a single dose and attached to a fine needle for one-time use. It is virtually impossible to re-use (e.g. by substance abusers).

Aside from the details about use of the injector – after shaking well, vertically, air bubble up, needle downward, subcutaneous administration into the abdomen or anterior thigh over 7 to 10 seconds (see http://www.medicines.org.uk/emc/medicine/27798) – nearly everything about Depo-Provera also applies

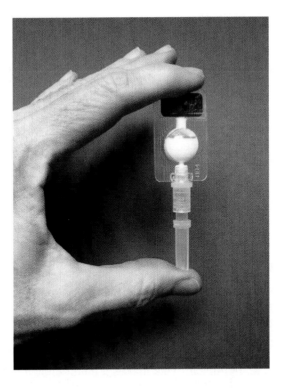

Figure 13
Sayana® Press DMPA for subcutaneous (sc) use. (Courtesy of Professor Anne MacGregor and Colin Parker of Durbin PLC.) (Note: bubble of air above the solution which is then given vertically by subcutaneous injection, into the anterior thigh or abdomen, slowly over 5 to 7 seconds.)

to Sayana Press. The subcutaneous route:

- Is advantageous in gross obesity.
- Minimizes deep haematoma risk for those on anticoagulants, but
- Has the risk of local skin problems (p. 89) – which can be minimised by varying the injection sites.
- Allows for simple self-injection (approved in late 2015); it is suggested that after training women be issued with doses for one year at a time.

This last property makes it more practical to implement for DMPA **the elimination of routine follow-up visits** (that is aside from the 2-yearly discussion visit that all users should have [p. 92]). The WHO and the FSRH now recommend, instead, a truly **'open house' policy** for all healthy, normotensive users of hormonal contraceptives, including, along with these injectables, all the CHCs, POPs, Nexplanon®, and IUCs. However, it must genuinely be the case that users who have any concerns about their method at any time after its initiation are seen promptly on request.

MECHANISM OF ACTION AND EFFECTIVENESS

DMPA is one of the most effective among the reversible methods (see Table 1), with a 'perfect use' failure rate of 0.2 (2 in 1000) in the first year of use (see Table 1). It functions primarily by causing anovulation, backed by effects on the cervical mucus similar to those of the POP and COC, as backup. A high initial blood level is achieved, declining over the next 3 months, but with much individual variation, staying above the level to inhibit ovulation for much longer in some women. Women in the latter group take longer to regain their fertility on ceasing DMPA (p. 95).

Higher body weight, more than 100 kg, or a BMI greater than 40 appears to confer an increased risk of failure with DMPA, whether intramuscular or subcutaneous. Consider shortening the injection interval.

Potential drug interactions

Contrary to previous advice, given that it has been shown that the liver ordinarily clears the blood reaching it completely of the drug – and enzyme inducers obviously cannot increase clearance beyond 100 per cent – there is no requirement to shorten the injection interval. This applies to many patients taking such drugs for epilepsy and even to users of the most powerful enzyme inducer, rifampicin. This makes it a first-choice option for many.

However, long-term users of anti-epileptic or anti-retroviral drugs that are enzyme inducing are at risk of osteopenia, osteoporosis and fractures, especially if they have other risk factors such as inadequate sun exposure. The National Institute for Health and Care Excellence (NICE) advises vitamin D supplementation for such women. Therefore, although DMPA has the maintained efficacy advantage just highlighted, the possibility that DMPA may further lower bone density (pp. 91–2) means that other options may need to be considered by such women, especially if they are immobilized for long periods or with other risk factors.

Starting routines – timing of the first injection
- In menstruating women, the first injection should ideally be given on day 1, but it can be given up to day 5 of the cycle; if given later than day 5 (see the earlier discussion), advise 7 days of extra precautions.
- If a woman is taking a COC or POP or the DSG POP up to the day of injection, give the injection any time, with no added precautions.
- Post partum (when the woman is not breastfeeding) or after a second-trimester abortion, the first injection should normally be at about day 21, and if later with added precautions for 7 days. If later and still amenorrhoeic, pregnancy risk must be excluded (can use the 'ploy' of pp. 160–1).

Earlier use just after delivery has been reported to lead to prolonged heavy bleeding, but it is sometimes clinically justified.
- During lactation, if DMPA is chosen, it is best given at 6 weeks.
- Lactation is not inhibited at all. The dose to the infant is small, and believed to be entirely harmless beyond 6 weeks.
- After miscarriage or a first-trimester abortion: injection on the day, or after expulsion of fetus if a medical procedure was used. If the injection is given beyond the fifth day, advise 7 days' extra precautions.

Overdue injections of DMPA with continuing sexual intercourse

How best to deal with these issues has caused much debate. The *normal* frequency for both intramuscular and subcutaneous injections is now accepted as every 13 weeks, so 12 weeks plus 7 days is not 'late'. The FSRH now defines an overdue injection that requires EC with sexual exposure as 14 weeks plus 1 day. That DMPA, unlike all other methods, cannot be stopped once given poses a problem, despite little evidence, fortunately, that it is harmful to a pregnancy.

The following box summarizes my own (JG) suggested protocol, modified from FSRH advice in their 2014 Guidance document (Table 4 of the Guidance; URL given on p. 83):

Protocol for overdue intramuscular or subcutaneous injection – beyond 91 days (13 weeks)
If a DMPA user has truly abstained ever since the due date, however late the injection, just give the next one and advise 7 days of added contraception.
If, however, there has been continuing unprotected sexual intercourse (UPSI):
A. **From day 92 until day 98 (the end of the 14th week: give the injection** and, optionally, the cautious advice (JG) to use added contraception during the next 7 days. Pregnancy testing is not indicated.
B. **Beyond day 99 (beyond the end of the 14th week), with earliest UPSI only up to 5 days before:**
- Assumption is that sex up to end of week 14 is protected. Offer EC and if hormonal, LNG EC is preferred (pp. 141–2). Then either:
  - Use the 'ploy' detailed on p. 161 (i.e. 'bridge' with well-taken DSG POP or a CHC (plus usual initial extra precautions) until next injection, to be given *if* pregnancy test is negative at 3 weeks since last UPSI).
  - Or, could give DMPA, provided a negative pregnancy test on the day and without the preliminary bridge (caution: injections are not removable [p. 89]), expecting renewed efficacy after 7 days.
- Unless the EC is by copper IUD, advise all to abstain or use condoms for 7 days following the hormonal EC (by LNG) plus injection.

C. Beyond end of 14th week with multiple UPSI episodes since day 99 including more than 5 days ago:
- Do a pregnancy test on the day. If negative can use the 'ploy' as above, but, with respect to EC: no EC method should be given if the sexual history suggests the possibility of an already implanted pregnancy. Beware, there is no simple clinical way to relate the timing of any EC to ovulation or fertilization. If hormonal EC chosen, LNG EC is preferred because, additionally, there is more evidence than for UPA that it would not harm an early conception, should there be inadvertent exposure of it to the EC method.
- Given a negative pregnancy test, the next DMPA injection may be given (without or possibly with LNG EC), provided the woman accepts an unquantified but small risk to any possible conception plus DMPA's lack of 'removeability'.

Using clinical judgement regarding implantation, in both situations B and C, on a case-by-case basis (see pp. 136–7), insertion of a copper IUD as EC may be appropriate and may sometimes lead the woman to switch to it for the long term. See Table 4 of the FSRH Guidance document on injectables for more – the URL for it is on p. 83. In all the foregoing circumstances, counsel the woman regarding possible failure and the need for a check pregnancy test if there is doubt.

What should *not* happen is for the woman with ongoing UPSI who is very late with her injection just to be told to go away until she has her next period because this may never come!

Note: DMPA may always be given early, after 10 weeks (FSRH); indeed, the earliest could be after the decline in peak blood levels at 8 weeks after a previous dose (JG, unlicensed, p. 165).

ADVANTAGES AND INDICATIONS

DMPA has obvious contraceptive benefits, but it also shares most of the non-contraceptive benefits of the COC described earlier, including protection against pelvic infection and endometrial cancer. Few metabolic changes have been described.

Indications for DMPA
Main indications
- The woman's desire for a highly effective method that is independent of intercourse and unaffected by enzyme inducers, and when other options are contraindicated or disliked.

- A past history of ectopic pregnancy or, as with all other progestogen-only methods, of past thrombosis or increased risk (e.g. for effective contraception while waiting for major or leg surgery). (The DSG POP is another option here.)

Non-contraceptive indications
- Endometriosis.
- Past symptomatic functional cysts.
- Sickle cell anaemia: reduces pain of sickle cell crises.
- Epilepsy, in which it often reduces the frequency of seizures.
- Menstrual problems may benefit (variably), if amenorrhoeic.

PROBLEMS AND DISADVANTAGES

Possibly its main disadvantage is unique among available contraceptives, that it is impossible to stop (i.e. to take the injection out again once given, e.g. inadvertently in pregnancy). Side effects may be for the duration, for 3 months, maybe more. It is *unfair* not to mention this fact in advance.

Side effects of DMPA, summarized
- Irregular, sometimes prolonged, bleeding and/or spotting (see the next box) – 'structured information' about this, at the start and repeated, has been shown to reduce discontinuation by 12 months. This is probably because perseverance so often leads to amenorrhoea (70 per cent by 1 year), which can be highly acceptable once it is understood that 'periods don't have any excretory function or health benefits'.
- Amenorrhoea* – a good side effect, but not always so seen.
- Delayed return of fertility – something to warn about (see later).
- Weight gain – a Cochrane review found a mean weight gain of about 3 kg at 2 years. However, some users, especially if their initial BMI was more than 30, gain considerably more than this – again, forewarn!
- Some concern regarding reduced bone density – (see later).
- There are reports of 'minor side effects' such as acne, headache, alopecia, hot flushes, mood change, and loss of libido, yet there is no hard evidence of a causal association with these. With respect to libido loss, the link at times with vaginal dryness or flushes suggests lowered estrogen levels as a factor in individual cases – and clinically finding another effective method may often improve all these symptoms.
- Injection site problems:
  - Haematoma if DMPA is given intramuscularly: rare, more common if the patient is anticoagulated and if so, use subcutaneous DMPA.
  - Infection with either route; also rare.
- *But* skin changes were noted in as many as 9 per cent of self-injecting users of the subcutaneous route and included induration, scarring and atrophy.

*It is helps to say 'there is no blood coming away because there is no blood there *to* come away'.

Bone density and related issues

Most DMPA users have estradiol (E_2) levels similar to the early to mid-follicular phase, but they are decidedly low for some women in the fertile years. The question is, does prolonged hypo-estrogenism in some women through use of DMPA lead, by analogy with premature menopause, to added risk of bone density loss or frank osteoporosis; or possibly arterial disease in those already predisposed, such as smokers?

Arterial disease

Despite negatively affecting HDL cholesterol, studies, including by WHO (1998), continue to be generally reassuring with respect to arterial as well as venous circulatory disease. A 1999 cohort study from Thailand found no difference in BP between IUD users and DMPA users after 10 years.

Bone mineral density

After more than 30 years of research, there remains uncertainty – not about the variably low follicular-phase E_2 levels that are found in DMPA users, but about their implications for bone health. We know that:

- Mean bone mineral density (BMD) is lower in DMPA users than in controls in cross-sectional comparisons, including among women older than 45 years, but not in ex-users post-menopausally.
- This finding is unconnected to the bleeding pattern (it may or may not occur in women experiencing either amenorrhoea or irregular bleeding).
- It increases again toward baseline on discontinuation in all age groups (suggestive that this loss is E_2 related and a real effect – but also very reassuring for reversibility). There is no proven risk of actual DMPA-related fractures.
- From limited evidence, the BMD in adolescent DMPA users is lower than in controls. This has raised the concern that normal peak bone mass may not be fully achieved if DMPA were used during teenage years. On the positive side for teens, however, is the evidence of reversibility (last bulleted item) and the fact that bone density does not finally peak until age 25 years. Having a general policy of switching from 3-monthly DMPA to a 3-yearly implant as soon as teens achieve amenorrhoea with the former (which is often in less than a year) will also address this concern (see the later protocol).
- Long-term DMPA-using women examined after menopause versus lifetime never users have not been shown to differ in bone density, again suggesting possible recovery of bone mass after stopping DMPA.

Based on the foregoing, UKMEC therefore simply states that DMPA is classified as WHO 2 for adolescents and for women older than 45 years.

How long to use DMPA (FSRH Guidance)?

Protocols for choice and duration of use of DMPA
First, if there is known osteopenia or osteoporosis, or if strong risk factors for osteoporosis already exist, DMPA is WHO 4. Examples of the latter:
- Long-term systemic corticosteroid treatment.
- Secondary amenorrhoea, resulting from e.g. anorexia nervosa or marathon running.
- An untreated malabsorption syndrome (e.g. gluten enteropathy).

However, the category could become WHO 3 if the risk factor has ceased, the young woman is obtaining sufficient estrogen either naturally during

---

normal cycling or as ethinylestradiol (EE) through the COC, or there is a scan (rarely indicated) showing good BMD.

- Under age 18, despite the foregoing concern that it may prevent achievement of peak bone mass, DMPA is WHO 2; hence FSRH Guidance confirms that it may be used as a first-line method after other methods have been discussed and considered unsuitable or unacceptable.
- After age 45 years, DMPA is also WHO 2 (because of the possibility of incipient ovarian failure and also because methods without this concern are available, such as the old-type POP, which would be equally effective at this age). After age 50, DMPA is WHO 3 (JG): the FSRH also supports continuation in well-counselled cases.

If the method is now chosen:

- DMPA remains a highly effective, safe and 'forgettable' method, usable by almost any woman in the childbearing years.
- Women should be informed that there may be a small loss of BMD, but this is usually recovered after discontinuation.
- In short, DMPA should now be presented as primarily a method for short- to medium-term use, after which switching to another long-term method such as an implant would be usual.
- There should be planned a regular 2-yearly discussion and individualized review of alternatives, but without blood tests or any imaging. Those tests (e.g. BMD scanning) are not a routine part of the protocol.
- At one of these 2-yearly discussions, usefully based on the Family Planning Association's leaflet *Your Contraceptive Choices,* many women will therefore choose to switch from DMPA to another long-acting method (e.g. to Nexplanon*, a copper IUD or the IUS) after 2, 4, or 6 years or after age 50 years to a POP. However:
- If instead the woman wishes to use DMPA for longer, it is as always her right to decide to do so, on the 'informed user-chooser' basis, after coun-selling about the uncertainty.
- It happens that African-Caribbean women have, genetically, higher BMD levels, as do obese women, so the provider may be more comfortable if these women wish to use DMPA for a longer duration than others.

*Practical advantages of this particular switch are as follows:
–The implant can be 'sold' as being essentially the same as their existing DMPA but with an injection every 3 years rather than every 3 months.
–There is a strong clinical impression that if the DMPA user has amenorrhoea, this reduces the risk of unacceptable bleeding when the implant is inserted – at least for the first year.
–The implant can be inserted at a time that suits everyone rather than having to be in the first 5 days of the cycle (see p. 101).

When all is said and done, the safety issue of osteoporosis with DMPA is in reality less than the widely accepted and rare yet real risk of lethal complica-tions of EE, within CHCs.

Are there not similar bone density concerns with long-term Nexplanon®?

There are not. The data are reassuring so far: in a non-randomized comparative study described below, after 2 years bone densities were remarkably similar among Nexplanon users and copper IUD users. By analogy, because the well-taken DSG POP is a bit like 'oral Nexplanon', there are no worries to date with the former – nor with any IUS, whose amenorrhoeic action is primarily at the end-organ level (the endometrium).

CONTRAINDICATIONS

These are similar to contraindications to the POP (JG's opinion) but affected by the higher dose and lack of immediate reversibility of DMPA.

Absolute contraindications to DMPA (WHO 4)
- Current osteopenia or osteoporosis on scan or severe risk factor(s) for osteoporosis, as noted earlier, including long-term corticosteroid treatment (>5 mg prednisolone/day).
- Any serious adverse effect of COCs not certainly related solely to the estrogen content (e.g. liver adenoma or cancer – although UKMEC classifies these as WHO 3).
- Recent breast cancer not yet clearly in remission (see later).
- History of acute porphyria (progestogens as well as estrogens are believed capable of precipitating these episodes, 1 per cent of attacks are fatal, and the injection is not 'removable').
- Hypersensitivity to any component.
- Actual or possible pregnancy.

WHO 3 conditions for DMPA
- Factors suggesting high risk of osteoporosis but normal or minimally reduced BMD on bone scan.
- Current ischaemic heart disease, severe arterial diseases including stroke (because of the foregoing evidence about low estrogen levels coupled with reports of lowered HDL cholesterol) and current VTE.
- Diabetes with any evidence of tissue damage or of more than 20 years' duration, also SLE with positive or unknown antiphospholipid antibodies. (Reasons given at the last bullet.)
- Familial hyperlipidaemias (other progestogen-only methods than DMPA such as the POP or the DSG POP are preferred).

- Breast cancer, in complete remission (after 5 years according to UKMEC). However, a POP or LNG-IUS would be preferable (lower dose, more reversible).
- Severe liver disease (acute viral hepatitis, decompensated cirrhosis).
- Undiagnosed genital tract bleeding until cause established.

WHO 2 conditions for DMPA *(usually posing negligible concerns)*
- Women younger than 18 or older than 45 years of age are at most only WHO 2 with respect to the bones (see earlier).
- History of VTE, any predisposition to VTE.
- Obesity, although further weight gain is not inevitable (see later).
- Hypertension, controlled on treatment.
- Hyperlipidaemias other than familial type (take advice).
- Strong family history of breast cancer – UKMEC says WHO 1 for this.
- Known *BRCA* mutation present.
- Cervical cancer or cervical intraepithelial neoplasia (CIN) awaiting treatment.
- Active liver disease: compensated cirrhosis, with moderately abnormal liver function.
- Gallbladder disease.
- Cholestasis history, CHC related.
- Porphyrias other than the acute intermittent variety.
- Bleeding tendency or any anti-coagulant therapy. The intramuscular route (Depo-Provera) carries a small risk of deep haematoma in the muscle, so this positively indicates use of subcutaneous DMPA, as Sayana Press. Nexplanon, which is inserted superficially, anterior to all major blood vessels, is also suitable.
- Breastfeeding less than 6 weeks post-partum.
- Past severe endogenous depression (UKMEC says WHO 1).
- Undiagnosed genital tract bleeding.
- Planning a pregnancy in the near future.
- Unwillingness to cope with prospect of irregularity or absence of periods – sometimes connected with cultural or religious taboos.

COUNSELLING

Aside from taking account of the WHO eligibility factors noted earlier, four main practical points must be made to prospective users:

- The effects, whether wanted (contraceptive) or unwanted, are not reversible for the duration of the injection: this fact is unique among current contraceptives.
- Weight gain, although no study has proved causation by any other hormonal contraceptives, is uniquely real with DMPA. It is believed to be caused by increased appetite, so it is useful (and can really work) to

advise a pre-emptive plan to start taking extra exercise as well as watching diet. It may help some women's decision making that women who are not already overweight put on significantly less than those who are.

- Irregular, sometimes prolonged, bleeding may be a problem, but the outlook is good (see earlier).
- **Conception is commonly delayed after the last dose**. There is a median delay of 9 months since the last injection, which is of course only around 6 months after cessation of the method. However, in some women it could be well over 1 year, and all women should be warned of that possibility. A comparative study in Thailand showed that almost 95 per cent of previously fertile users had conceived by 28 months after their last injection. *So there is no evidence of permanent infertility*, in any age group, including teenagers with treatment initiated early post-menarche. With respect to continuing post-DMPA amenorrhoea:
  - If conception is not wanted, alternative contraception must begin from about 13 weeks since the last injection.
  - If conception is wanted, spontaneous ovulation can be anticipated in most cases: if not, refer for investigation with or without treatment at about 12 months after the last injection.

FOLLOW-UP

Aside from ensuring the injections take place at the correct intervals, follow-up is primarily advisory and supportive:

- Prolonged or too frequent bleeding is managed as already described.
- BP is normally checked initially, but there is absolutely no need for it to be taken before each dose because studies fail to show any hypertensive effect. As routine follow-up, supported by FSRH Guidance, 2-yearly visits mainly for discussion of alternatives is enough (p. 92), so long as there is always that essential 'open house' for any DMPA user who has problems. Those who self-administer DMPA subcutaneously should have an opportunity to discuss any concerns annually, when they have their prescription renewed (see p. 92).

Contraceptive implants

The most common implants worldwide contain a progestogen in a slow-release carrier, made either of polydimethylsiloxane, as in Jadelle® or Sino-implant® (not available in the United Kingdom) with two implants, or ethylene vinyl acetate (EVA), as in Nexplanon® otherwise known in some locations as Implanon NXT®, a single rod (Figure 14).

They are excellent examples of LARCs, with the ideal 'forgettable' default state, yet rapid reversibility.

MECHANISM OF ACTION, ADMINISTRATION AND EFFECTIVENESS

Nexplanon, formerly known as Implanon, works primarily by ovulation inhibition, supplemented mainly by the usual sperm-blocking mucus effect. It is a single 40-mm rod, just 2 mm in diameter, containing 68 μg of etonogestrel – the chief active metabolite of desogestrel – and so has much in common with a well-taken DSG POP. This is dispersed in an EVA matrix and covered by a 0.06-mm rate-limiting EVA membrane. The rod now also contains barium sulphate, so it can be imaged by X-ray studies but it remains bio-equivalent to Implanon, with the same release rate and 3-year licensed duration of action.

See the Faculty of Sexual and Reproductive Healthcare (FSRH) Guidance at: www.fsrh.org/pdfs/CEUGuidanceProgestogenOnlyImplants.pdf, and www.fsrh.org/pages/Letter_of_Competence_SDI.asp for more on training for Nexplanon. The latter URL describes the requirements for nurses or doctors for electronic sexual and reproductive health (eSRH) training, model-arm and live training in insertion and removal techniques and the maintenance of expertise.

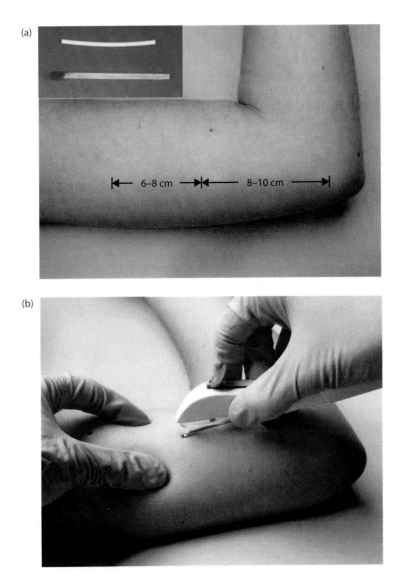

(a)

|← 6–8 cm →|← 8–10 cm →|

(b)

Figure 14
Nexplanon, showing (a) positioning and marking up of the arm and (b) subsequent use of inserter system. (Courtesy of Professor Anne MacGregor.)

Nexplanon – the main points summarized
- Nexplanon is inserted subdermally but very superficially under the skin over the biceps, medially in the upper arm, under local anaesthesia, from a dedicated sterile pre-loaded applicator by a simple one-handed injection-and-withdrawal technique. Note the positioning of the recipient's arm

(see Figure 14). The provider should be seated so as to see the progress of the needle, following the instructions provided with the product.

- Current teaching, following the revised Summary of Product Characteristics (SPC), is to insert away from and usually anterior to the groove between the triceps and biceps, hence superficial to the biceps muscle and well away from the neurovascular bundle.
- Although this implant is much easier than Norplant® was to insert or to remove, specific training is essential and cannot be obtained from any book. In the United Kingdom, the best training for nurses or doctors is obtainable through the FSRH to obtain their Letter of Competence (LOC) in sub-dermal implants (SDIs). Details at: www.fsrh.org/pages/Training.asp
- After an initial phase of several weeks of giving higher blood levels, Nexplanon delivers almost constant low daily levels of the hormone, for a recommended duration of use of 3 years.
- In the pre-marketing trials, Nexplanon had the unique distinction of a zero failure rate. The 'perfect use' failure rate is now estimated as about 5 in 10 000 insertions (see Table 1). Therefore, because 'user failures' are improbable it shares the status with the LNG implants of most effective reversible contraceptives ever devised.
- Most of the 'failures' that have been reported either had had the insertion during a conception cycle or were failures to insert at all. Almost all the later failures were related to enzyme-inducer drugs.
- Effect of body mass? In the international studies, serum levels tended to be lower in overweight women, but in the post-marketing study, failures attributed to high body mass were not reported. It is unclear whether this is because providers have been offering other methods to grossly over-weight women or replacing implants early as advised by the SPC – or a function of the 'margin of safety' of this incredibly effective method.
- However, clinically, it is clear that this finding should not deter provid-ers from offering Nexplanon to overweight women as a medically safer option than any CHC (especially Evra®), with respect to VTE risk.
- Reversibility is normally simple by removal of the implant, with almost immediate effect.

MAINTAINING EFFECTIVENESS

The main causes of failure

All are rare, but include the following:

- Insertion during a conception cycle – discussed later (p. 101).
- Failure to insert at all – should now be vanishingly rare, given the new inserter technology plus the advice (if followed) that both provider and user always palpate the Nexplanon *in situ* just after insertion.
- Enzyme-inducing drugs.

What about body weight?

Is this relevant? See the seventh bullet in the previous box. The SPC states:

> The contraceptive effect of Nexplanon is related to the plasma levels of etonogestrel, which are inversely related to body weight, and decrease with time after insertion… It cannot be excluded that the contraceptive effect in these women during the third year of use may be lower than for women of normal weight. HCPs [healthcare providers] may therefore consider earlier replacement of the implant in heavier women.

The word 'consider' there is unclear for providers: my own practice based on anecdotes of failure would be to discuss earlier replacement with a young fertile woman with weight well over 100 kg, if she also began to cycle regularly in the third year (suggesting reliance only on the mucus effect, p. 96).

Enzyme-inducer drug treatment

The SPC states that hepatic enzyme inducers may lower the blood levels of etonogestrel and there have certainly been associated failures, though without confirmatory interaction studies. Women on short-term treatment are advised to use a barrier method in addition and (because reversal of enzyme induction always takes time) for 28 days thereafter. During long-term treatment, because enzyme-inducer drug users do so well with DMPA or an IUD or IUS, these are definitely the preferred choices.

ADVANTAGES AND INDICATIONS

The main indication is the woman's desire for a highly effective yet at all times rapidly reversible method, without the finality of sterilization, which is independent of intercourse, especially when other options are contraindicated or disliked.

- Above all, it provides efficacy and convenience – if the bleeding pattern suits, it is a 'forgettable' contraceptive.
- It has a long duration of action with one treatment (3 years) – a 'selling point' when switching from DMPA – and high continuation rates.
- There is no initial peak dose given orally to the liver.
- Blood levels are low and fairly steady, rather than fluctuating (as with the POP) or initially too high (as with each dose of injectables); this, with the previous point, means that metabolic changes are few and believed to be negligible.
- Nexplanon is estrogen-free and therefore definitely usable if there is a history of VTE (WHO category 2).
- Median systolic and diastolic BP were unchanged in trials for up to 4 years.

- Because it is an anovulant, special indications include past ectopic pregnancy.
- The effects are rapidly reversible, an advantage over DMPA that is worth emphasizing. After removal, serum etonogestrel levels are undetectable after 4 days, so return of fertility must be assumed to be almost immediate.

CONTRAINDICATIONS

Contraindications are very similar to those to use of the DSG POP because Nexplanon is an anovulant, yet, unlike DMPA, immediately reversible – and they contain essentially the same progestogen.

Absolute contraindications (WHO 4) for Nexplanon
- Any serious adverse effect of COCs not certainly related solely to the estrogen (e.g. liver adenoma or cancer: UKMEC is more permissive, WHO 3).
- Recent breast cancer not yet clearly in remission (see later).
- Known or suspected pregnancy.
- Hypersensitivity to any component.

WHO 3 conditions for Nexplanon
- Current ischaemic heart disease, severe arterial diseases including stroke.
- Sex steroid–dependent cancer, including breast cancer, when in complete remission (UKMEC states WHO 4 until 5 years, then WHO 3). Agreement of the relevant hospital consultant should be obtained and the woman's autonomy respected: record that she understands it is unknown whether progestogen may alter the recurrence risk (either way).
- Severe liver disease (acute viral hepatitis, decompensated cirrhosis).
- Acute porphyria, if there is a history of actual attack triggered by sex hormones (my view, because progestogens as well as estrogens are believed capable of precipitating these attacks, and 1 per cent of such attacks are fatal). Otherwise, the history of acute porphyria is WHO 2.
- Undiagnosed genital tract bleeding until cause established.
- Enzyme-inducer drugs – although very exceptionally, in my view, an added DSG POP daily may be taken, off licence (p. 165). Another LARC such as an injectable, IUD or IUS would be a better choice.

TIMING OF NEXPLANON INSERTION

- In the woman's natural cycle, day 1 to 5 is the usual timing; if any day later than day 5 (provided no sexual exposure up to that day) is chosen, recommend additional contraception for 7 days.
- Helpfully, if a woman is on COC, POP or the DSG POP or DMPA, the implant can normally be inserted at any time, overlapping with the other method, with no added precautions.

Clinical implications

Insertions only during the foregoing tiny natural-cycle window are a logistic nightmare! There is also pressure on providers, when women arrive later in the cycle without 'believable abstinence' or full security about condom use, to insert the implant anyway.

So a useful practical tip is to actively recommend, as the normal routine (as also recommended for insertion of IUSs) at counselling, the use or re-use of an anovulant method (i.e. one of those in the second bullet point in the insertion box), to continue until the Nexplanon insertion.

An extension of this concept is to recommend to Nexplanon requesters that they defer the insertion until they have achieved amenorrhoea through

DMPA injections, as many or as few as they need to have stopped all bleeding for (say) 60 days – and insert the implant only after that. This often occurs after two to four injections (p. 89). Clinical experience suggests (although we badly need the results of a planned clinical trial to prove the point) that, as with insertions during amenorrhoea post partum, this will reduce the risk of unacceptable bleeding thereafter.

Timing in non-cycling states
- Following delivery (not breastfeeding) or second-trimester abortion, insertion on about day 21 is recommended, or if later with additional contraception for 7 days. If later and still amenorrhoeic, pregnancy risk should be excluded, often by 'bridging' first with a Pill method for 3 weeks, followed by a negative pregnancy test result (p. 161).
- If breastfeeding, insert ideally on day 21 with no need for added contraception for 7 days. Reassurance can be given that the implant can safely be used in lactation – the infant will receive approximately 0.2 per cent of the estimated maternal dose.
- Following first-trimester abortion, immediate insertion is best
  - On the day of surgically induced abortion or the second part of a medical abortion.
  - Or up to 5 days later.
  - If more than 5 days later, an added method such as condom use is recommended for 7 days.
- To follow any other effective contraceptive (CHC, POP, DMPA, IUD, IUS), it is often best to overlap the methods by at least 7 days so there is no loss of protection between methods and no need to discuss supplementary condom use.
- To replace a previous Nexplanon after 3 years, the new one may be inserted through the same removal incision but along a different track, with additional local anaesthetic and ensuring that the needle is inserted to its full length.

COUNSELLING AND ONGOING SUPERVISION

Always explain the likely changes to the bleeding pattern and the possibility of 'hormonal' side effects (see later). This discussion should, as always, be backed by a good leaflet, such as the Family Planning Association (FPA) handout, and well documented.

No treatment-specific follow-up is necessary (including no need for BP checks). The SPC recommends the option of one follow-up visit at 3 months. More important is an explicit 'open-house' policy, so the woman knows she can return at any time to discuss possible side effects and their treatment (see later), without any provider pressure to persevere if the woman really wants the implant removed (the service standard for the maximum wait for removal should be no more than 2 weeks). If the removal is for unacceptable bleeding, the most common reason, consider offering an LNG-IUS to follow. Jaydess® usually produces bleeding that is light and regular (p. 123).

Bleeding problems

- Experience shows that around 55 per cent of women have a bleeding pattern that, although often irregular, is acceptably light and infrequent. Forewarning with reassurance in advance that this is not harmful is crucial for achieving low removal rates.
- About 20 per cent of women develop amenorrhoea by 1 year, and with forewarning and reassurance most of these will persevere.
- About 25 per cent have frequent or prolonged bleeding and spotting. Whatever is experienced in the first 3 months is broadly predictive of future bleeding patterns.

Clinical management of unacceptable bleeding

With reassurance, most women are happy to accept one of the patterns in the first two groups described earlier. For the third group, perseverance beyond 3 months is rewarded less often than with DMPA (or the IUS). After eliminating unrelated causes for the bleeding, such as *Chlamydia* infection or other relevant items in the crucial "D" Checklist on p. 59:

- The best short-term treatment is cyclical estrogen therapy. The current annoying bleeding usually stops in a few days, and then it is preferable (JG) to produce those 'pharmacological curettages' (i.e. episodes of withdrawal bleeding), on a similar basis to the regimen for DMPA (p. 90). This may most easily be provided by three cycles of any COC containing 20 μg or, if necessary, 30 μg of ethinylestradiol (EE), after which the bleeding may (or sometimes may not!) become acceptable. This plan should be explained in advance to the woman, who should also understand the uncertainty whether it will 'work' for her. Courses may be repeated if an acceptable bleeding pattern does not follow. Or,
- If the foregoing approach fails or the woman has a WHO 4 contraindication to EE, an alternative based on data extrapolated from studies with LNG implants is to try a short course of mefenamic acid 500 mg up to three times daily. A 5–7 day course usually stops a prolonged bleed.
- Some clinicians report that giving, empirically, an added DSG POP tablet daily has been successful – enough times to be worth a try.

We badly need good RCTs to establish the value or otherwise of the foregoing regimens. Personally, I (JG) favour the previously stated policy of attempting to pre-empt annoying bleeding problems by creating amenorrhoea first, using DMPA – although whether this approach works long term (rather than just in early months) and raises continuation rates also needs confirmation.

> **Minor side effects**
>
> Reported in frequency order, minor side effects were:
> - Acne (but this also sometimes improved!).
> - Headache.
> - Abdominal pain.
> - Breast pain.
> - 'Dizziness'.
> - Mood changes (depression, emotional lability).
> - Libido decrease.
> - Hair loss.

There is no scientific proof of a causal link between the implant and any of the symptoms in the previous box – including the often-alleged problems of weight gain, mood change and loss of libido. However, users should always be 'met where they are' – and if they are convinced that their symptom is related to the implant, and is unacceptable, they need to be actively helped to find an alternative acceptable method.

> **Local adverse effects**
>
> The following local adverse effects may also occur:
> - Infection of the site.
> - Expulsion.
> - Migration and difficult removal.
> - Scarring (very rare).

Bone mineral density

Because Nexplanon suppresses ovulation and does not supply any estrogen, the same questions as with DMPA arise over possible hypo-estrogenism. However, in a non-randomized comparative study, no estradiol or bone density differences in the means, ranges or standard errors were detected between 44 users of Nexplanon and 29 users of copper IUDs over 2 years, a finding that is reassuring, pending more data.

It appears that, despite its amazing efficacy through blocking luteinizing hormone (LH) surges and ovulation, the suppression of follicle-stimulating hormone (FSH) levels by Nexplanon is less, allowing generally higher follicular estrogen levels, than in (some) users of DMPA.

Reversibility and removal problems

Reversal is normally simple, with almost immediate effect. Under local anaesthesia, steady digital pressure on the palpable proximal end of the Nexplanon, after a 2-mm incision over the distal end, leads to delivery of that end of the rod; removal is completed by grasping it with mosquito forceps. As for insertion, removal training is crucial, using the 'model arm' and also live under supervision.

Removal problems can be minimized by good training in both insertion and removal techniques. Impalpable devices correlate with initially too deep insertion (possible even with the latest inserter). Beware particularly of the thin or very muscular woman with very little subcutaneous tissue. Insertion can easily permit a segment of the rod to enter an arm muscle, with deep migration following.

A plain X-ray film will display a 'lost' Nexplanon, but removal of the device may need to be under ultrasound control. The manufacturer (MSD) has a UK panel of expert removers, so it is recommended to contact them in the first instance for advice and help in such cases.

Intrauterine contraceptives (IUCs) are of two distinct types:

- Copper intrauterine devices (IUD or IUDs), in which the copper ion (the actual contraceptive) is released from a band or wire on a plastic carrier.
- The levonorgestrel (LNG)-releasing intrauterine systems (IUS or IUSs – generically), which release that progestogen: initially 20 µg daily from Mirena® or Levosert® and 14 µg from the smaller Jaydess®. In this book, LNG-IUS used unqualified will refer to the larger systems loaded with 52 mg LNG. The smaller system, which contains LNG 13.5 mg, will be referred to either as Jaydess or as the 13.5-mg LNG-IUS.

The latest (2015) very comprehensive Faculty of Sexual and Reproductive Healthcare (FSRH) Guidance can be accessed at www.fsrh.org/pdfs/CEUGuidanceIntrauterineContraception.pdf.

COPPER-BEARING DEVICES

'It is time to forgive the intrauterine device!'

This headline of an article says it all. Actually, there are well over 150 million users worldwide, but the lion's share is in just one country – China. It seems improbable that the difference between approximately 1 per cent of sexually active users in the United States or approximately 7 per cent in the United Kingdom and more than 20 per cent in France is explicable by some important differences among the French, the British and the US uterus. Do the Chinese and the French have something to teach the rest of the world?

In many countries, women in their late 30s have not been requesting IUDs because they were told by their mothers to avoid that method. This is unfortunate because in reality a woman in her later reproductive years with, say, two or three children, is the ideal user. The devices have changed over the years, but importantly she has, too – a parous cervical canal makes insertion easier, and commonly she also has less exposure to sexually transmitted infections (STIs) than in her youth (though nulliparae may also be good candidates for the method).

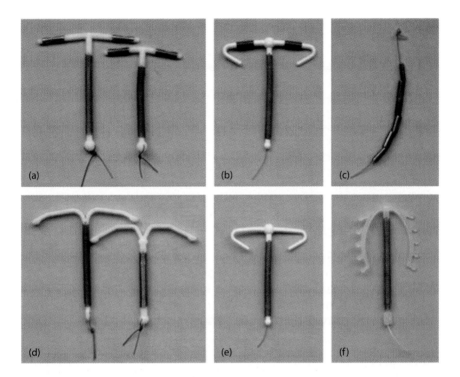

Figure 15
Copper intrauterine devices (IUDs). (a) TT 380 Slimline® (Durbin) and Mini TT 380 Slimline® (Durbin) with short stem. T-Safe Cu 380A QL® (Quick Load) (Williams). T-Safe 380A Capped® (Williams). (b) Flexi-T+380® (Durbin). (c) GyneFix Viz® (Williams & Durbin). (d) UT 380 Standard® (Durbin) and UT 380 Short® (Durbin) with short stem. Nova T380® (Bayer). Neo-Safe T380® (Williams). (e) Flexi-T 300® (Durbin) Cu-Safe T300® (Williams). (f) Multiload Cu375® (MSD) Load 375® (Durbin). (Courtesy of Professor Anne MacGregor, and Colin Parker of Durbin PLC.)

Some doctors are complying too readily with requests for male or female sterilization that originate partly from 'medical myths' about the intrauterine alternative. Leaving aside the significant advance represented by the IUSs, too few women know that the latest banded copper IUDs (Figure 15) can also be accurately described as 'reversible sterilization'.

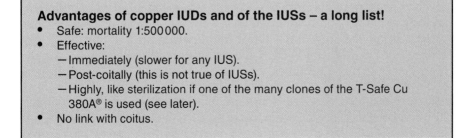

Advantages of copper IUDs and of the IUSs – a long list!
- Safe: mortality 1:500 000.
- Effective:
  - Immediately (slower for any IUS).
  - Post-coitally (this is not true of IUSs).
  - Highly, like sterilization if one of the many clones of the T-Safe Cu 380A® is used (see later).
- No link with coitus.

- No tablets to remember.
- Continuation rates are high and permitted duration of use can exceed 10 years.
- Reversible – and there is evidence that this is true even when the devices have been removed for one of the recognized complications.
- A systematic review (2002) found that copper IUDs may reduce the risk of both cancer of the endometrium and cervix. This is as yet unexplained, unlike the probable protective effect against endometrial cancer of the LNG-IUS (which, as Mirena, is licensed to protect the endometrium against the otherwise increased rate of this cancer in hormone replacement therapy [HRT] users).

Mechanism of action

- Appropriate studies indicate that copper IUDs operate primarily by preventing fertilization; the copper ion is toxic to sperm.
- Their effectiveness when inserted post-coitally shows that they act additionally to block implantation. However, when IUDs are *in situ* long term, this is a secondary or backup mechanism.

Clinical implication
- Because in any given cycle, this type of IUC may be working through the block of implantation, there is a small risk of 'iatrogenic' conception if a device is removed after mid-cycle, even if abstinence follows.
- Ideally, therefore, women should either use another method additionally from 7 days before planned device removal or, if this has not been the case, postpone removal until the next menses.
- If a device must be removed earlier, hormonal post-coital contraception may be indicated.

Choice of devices and effectiveness

In the United Kingdom, the 'gold standard' among IUDs for a parous woman without menstrual problems (if these are present, an IUS would be preferable) is a banded copper IUD (see Figure 15).

The nomenclature of the devices available is a nightmare! (see Figure 15): they include the generic T-Safe Cu 380A, with new variants with their copper bands sunk into the arms of the plastic frame, which are branded as TT 380 'Slimline'® or T-Safe Cu 380A QL 'Quick Load'® (these are available, respectively, from Durbin and FP Sales – see British National Formulary [BNF]).

In Sivin's Population Council randomized controlled trial, efficacy of this banded IUD type was statistically similar to that of the LNG-IUS. The cumulative failure rate of the CuT 380Ag® to 10 years was only 1.4 per 100 women (compare a mean rate of 1.8 per 100 women at 10 years after female sterilization in the American CREST study from 1996). There were no failures at all after year 5!

The banded copper device is therefore like 'reversible sterilization' – at least as performed in the United States before 1996. However, a World Health Organization (WHO) trial (referenced in FSRH Guidance, 2007) suggests that the LNG-IUS may be even more effective, and the US data of Table 1 (p. 9) show the same.

Important influence of age on effectiveness

Copper IUDs are much more effective in older women – largely because of declining fertility. After the age of 30 years, there is also a reduction in rates of expulsion and of pelvic inflammatory disease (PID) – the latter is believed not to be the result of resistance to infection of the older uterus but rather because the older woman is generally less exposed to the risk of infection (whether through her own lifestyle or that of her partner).

Advantages of one of the banded IUDs

The efficacy of the T-Safe Cu 380A in one randomized controlled trial was greater than that of the all-wire Nova T380®. It is licensed for 10 years, and the data support effectiveness until 12 years (even when fitted in women younger than 40 years; see later). However, the main advantage lies in the infrequency of re-insertions. Research in the past 50 years has so clearly shown the truth of both of the following slogans:

IUC Slogan 1
Insertion can be a factor in the causation of almost every category of IUC problems.

IUC Slogan 2
Most IUD- or IUS-related problems become less common with increasing duration of use.

Therefore, why would one ever use a 5-year device when a 10-year one will fit? Fewer insertions and the expected benefit from long-term use add up to 'banded is best!'

What if the woman is nulliparous?

Note that nulliparity *per se* is not a WHO category 4 for this method, despite the clinical practice of many doctors suggesting this! Indeed, after age 20 years, UKMEC classifies it as WHO 1/UKMEC 1. The T-Safe Cu 380A and its clones, the 'Slimline' and 'Quick Load', are not necessarily too large, but the first choice now for nulliparae is the Mini TT 380 Slimline® (Durbin), with reduced dimensions but exactly the same amount of copper. Therefore, it must be usable for the same 10-year minimum duration as the larger variant, and approval for this is being sought. Its 4.75 mm insertion tube is unfortunately no thinner, yet it usually passes readily through the nulliparous cervix, possibly after minimal dilation, and can be used for cavities sounding to as short as 5 cm.

Otherwise, for a comfortable and satisfactory fitting, one of the small wire-bearing IUDs with narrower insertion tubes may be better (see the options later), with the caveat of possibly reduced efficacy and a shorter duration of use (5 years).

When to use other IUDs (e.g. Nova T380 and its clones)

> **For emergency contraception – second-choice copper IUDs**
> The Nova T380/Neo-safe T 380®/UT 380 Standard® or the shorter UT 380 Short® may be appropriate if there are technical difficulties at the internal os because their inserter tube is only 3.6 mm wide – and the Short version will usefully fit any cavity more than 5 cm long (see Figure 15). A short-term emergency contraception (EC) option for such cases is the Flexi-T 300® with its 3.5-mm inserter tube and an easy push-in fitting technique with no separate plunger. However, it has a high expulsion rate, so the UT 380 Short – which also carries more copper and whose insertion tube is very nearly as thin – is a better bet, for potential longer use up to 5 years.

> **Difficult fittings**
> See pp. 130–2 for detailed clinical advice.
> * For long-term use, the Nova T380 or a 'clone' and the UT 380 Short (Nova T style but on a shorter stem, from Durbin) should usually be reserved for when the T-Safe Cu 380A or equivalent cannot be fitted, for some reason. The reason could be an unusually tight cervix or acute flexion of the uterus – rare in parous women but not uncommon in nulliparae.
> * There is also available the Flexi-T + 380®, on a slightly larger frame and with the advantage of bands on its sidearms but otherwise identical in shape. We need more data on this – sought but not so far forthcoming!
> * The Multiload IUDs, even the 375 thicker wire versions, were – in most of the randomized controlled trials – generally no better or less effective than the T-Safe Cu 380A, with no firm evidence of the reputed better expulsion rate.

When to use the banded but frameless GyneFix Viz®

This unique frameless device features a knot that is embedded by its special inserter system in the fundal myometrium (see Figure 15). Below the knot, its polypropylene thread bears six copper bands and locates them within the uterine cavity. Being frameless, it is less likely to cause uterine pain, and when correctly inserted it appears to rival the efficacy of the T-Safe Cu 380A. Unfortunately, in routine UK practice it was found to have a high (rather than the expected low) expulsion rate – and all users should be forewarned about the observed risk of unrecognized expulsion. Being able to feel the threads is particularly important with GyneFix Viz.

If it is available (by referral to someone trained in the specific insertion skills required), indications for GyneFix Viz include:
- Distorted cavity on ultrasound scan (if IUD is useable at all).
- A small uterine cavity sounding less than 6 cm (a rival and probably more available option if the uterus sounds to at least 5 cm is the UT 380 Short). Beware: short cavities are rare; one may have sounded only the cervix.
- Previous history of expulsion or removal of a framed device that was accompanied by excessive cramping, within hours or days of insertion.

Fortunately, because the names of copper IUDs are so confusing, from now onward all mentions of either 'IUD' or 'copper IUD' will refer, unless otherwise stated, only to the banded T-Safe Cu 380A or one of its 'clones'.

Main problems and disadvantages of copper IUDs

The main medical problems are listed in the following box and are dealt with in more detail thereafter. This is actually a remarkably short list as compared with the hormonal methods.

Possible problems with copper IUDs
1. Intrauterine pregnancy – hence its risks, including miscarriage.
2. Extrauterine pregnancy – because this is prevented less well than intrauterine (although the absolute risk is definitely reduced in population terms).
3. Expulsion – giving again the risks of pregnancy or miscarriage.
4. Perforation, with
   - Risks to bowel or bladder, and again
   - Risks of pregnancy.
5. Pelvic infection – as with item 2, the IUC is not causative, but it is not protective, either.
6. Malpositioning – which predisposes to items 1, 3 and 7.
7. Pain.
8. Bleeding, which can be
   - Increased amount.
   - Increased duration.

Note, clinically from foregoing summary box, that:

IUC Slogan 3 (see also Slogan 6)
Pain and bleeding in IUC users may signify a potentially dangerous
condition – a 'red flag' symptom until proved otherwise.

This means that all of the first six problems in the previous list need to be
excluded as diagnoses before pain and bleeding are ascribed simply to
being side effects of this method.

In situ conception

If the woman wishes to go on to full-term pregnancy, after a pelvic ultrasound
scan, the device should normally be removed – in the first trimester. This is
counter-intuitive, because one would think that this would increase the miscarriage rate. The truth is the reverse: for example, with *in situ* failures of the
Copper T 200 device, the normal rate of spontaneous abortion was 55 per
cent, dropping to 20 per cent if the device was removed. The woman should
of course be warned that an increased risk of miscarriage still remains.

Other clinical points
- If the woman is going to have a termination of her pregnancy, her IUD (or
  IUS) can be removed at the planned surgical procedure; however, it is
  safest to remove it before any medical abortion.
- If the threads are already missing when she is seen and other causes are
  excluded, aided by an ultrasound scan (see later): the pregnancy is at
  increased risk of
  − Second-trimester abortion (which could be infected).
  − Antepartum haemorrhage.
  − Premature labour.
- If the woman goes on to full-term pregnancy, it is essential to identify
  clearly the device in the products of conception. If it is not found, a post-
  partum X-ray study should be arranged in case the device is embedded
  or malpositioned or has perforated. There have been medico-legal cases,
  when this was not done, because of delayed diagnosis of a perforation,
  or unnecessary tests and treatments for 'infertility' when trying for a later
  wanted pregnancy, caused by a much earlier malpositioned IUC with no
  visible threads remaining *in situ,* ever since the original delivery.

There is no evidence of associated teratogenicity with conception during or
immediately after use of copper devices.

IUDs with 'lost threads'

This symptom of 'lost threads' links together points 1, 3, 4 and 6 in the box
on p. 111. There are at least six causes of this condition – three with and

three without pregnancy. An intra-abdominal IUC is just as useless at stopping pregnancy as one that has been totally expelled. More commonly, the woman is already pregnant, and the threads have been drawn up – or the device has altered its position *in situ.*

IUC Slogan 4
The woman with 'lost threads' is already pregnant until proven otherwise – moreover, even if not yet pregnant, she is likely to be unprotected and at risk of becoming pregnant.

'Lost threads' – six possible causes

Pregnant	Not pregnant
Unrecognized expulsion and pregnancy	Unrecognized expulsion and not yet pregnant
Perforation and pregnancy	Perforation and not yet pregnant
Device *in situ* and pregnancy	Device *in situ* and malpositioned or threads short (in uterus, if not found in cervical canal)

Diagnosis and management may involve some or all of the examinations and techniques shown in Figure 16. In this flow diagram, the later stages should follow referral to a specialist.

More about perforation
This is a general estimated risk for all IUCs of no more than about 1–2 per 1000 insertions, but the exact rate (as for expulsion) depends much less on the IUC design than on the skill of the clinician. Perforated devices should now almost always be removable at laparoscopy, but not as an emergency unless there is suspicion of bowel or vessel damage. See p. 129 re insertion in lactation.

Pelvic inflammatory disease and IUDs – what is the truth?
This is the great fear we all have about IUDs. Just as the Pill has been blamed for problems that we now know were caused by smoking, copper IUDs have been blamed for infections that were really acquired sexually (see the Chinese evidence, later).

Much of the anxiety derived from the Dalkon Shield disaster – but this was a unique device with a polyfilamentous thread, facilitating the transfer by capillary action of potential pathogens from the lower to the upper genital tract. Modern copper devices have a monofilamentous thread. They do not themselves cause infection.

However, they provide no protection against PID (in contrast to LNG-IUSs: which may protect slightly; see p. 125), and there is some suspicion that the

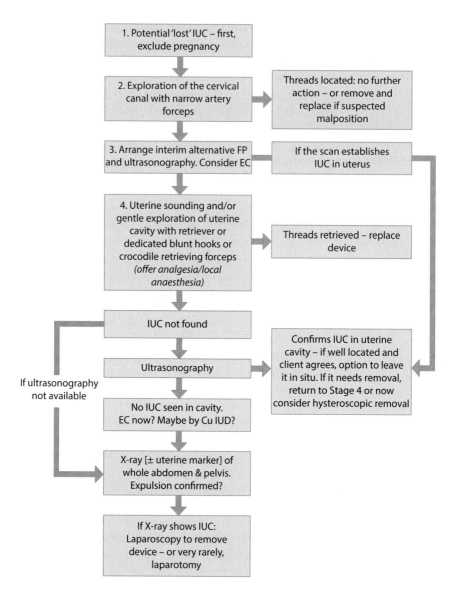

Figure 16
Management of 'lost' threads of IUCs (i.e. whether IUDs or IUSs).

infections that occur may perhaps be more severe as a result of the foreign body effect.

In a classic WHO study, Farley *et al.* (*Lancet* 1992;339:785–788) reported on a database from a number of WHO randomized controlled trials including approximately 23 000 insertions of copper IUDs or the

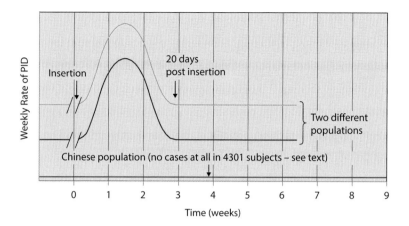

Figure 17
Schematic representation of main finding of World Health Organization (WHO) study of 22 908 intrauterine contraceptive (IUC) insertions (4301 in China) in Europe, Africa, Asia and the Americas (reference in text). Note that the weekly rate of pelvic inflammatory disease (PID) returns to the pre-insertion background rate for the population studied.

LNG-IUS, worldwide. In every country but one, the same pattern emerged (Figure 17):

- There was an IUD-associated increased risk of infection for 20 days after the insertion.
- However, the weekly infection rate 3 weeks after insertion went back to the same weekly rate as existed before insertion (i.e. the norm for that particular society).

In China, the one exception, there were no infections diagnosed at all in spite of 4301 insertions.

Interpretation
These findings are interpreted as follows:

- The post-insertion 'hump' of infections cannot be the result of poor insertion technique, restricted to doctors outside China.
- It is much more likely that, although the doctors in all the centres were searching for truly monogamous STI-free couples, they were successful in this search only in China (during the 1980s, when it is well recognized that China was practically an STI-free zone – China is no longer unique in this respect today).
- In the other countries, PID-causing organisms (especially *Chlamydia trachomatis*) are presumed to have been present – no cervical pre-screening being available at that time – in a proportion of the women. The process of insertion would interfere with natural defence mechanisms

(as has been confirmed when there is instrumentation in other contexts, such as therapeutic abortion).

- This would enable organisms to spread from the lower genital tract, where they had previously resided asymptomatically, into the upper genital tract, so causing the PID.

In summary, therefore:

> **IUC Slogan 5**
> The contraceptive devices, intrinsically, cannot be the cause of the PID that occurs in IUD and IUS users. (Otherwise, how improbable it is that there would have been 4301 Chinese users in the 1980s research and not a single reported attack!) Hence antibiotic cover is inappropriate if based just on the fact of an IUC insertion.

- The greatest infection risk is in the first 20 days, most probably caused by pre-existing carriage of STIs.
- Risk thereafter, as with pre-insertion, relates to the background risk of STIs (high in Africa, but so low in mainland China in the 1980s that it seems to have been absent in the study population).

> Therefore, the evidence-based policy should be that:
> - Elective IUC insertions and re-insertions should always occur through a 'Chinese cervix' (i.e. one that has been established to be pathogen-free), so hopefully eliminating the post-insertion infections shown in Figure 17.

> **Clinical implications for IUC insertion arrangements**
> - Prospective IUC users should always be verbally screened, meaning a good sexual history (p. 7). They need to know that they will need to use condoms, too, if the method is judged WHO 3 because of situational high STI risk – or even abandon this choice and use another method altogether.
> - Also – and this is the thorny one we all tend to leave out – 'Do you ever wonder if your partner has or is likely to have another sexual relationship?' (Reworded as appropriate, and always with the utmost tact.)
> - In populations with high prevalence of *C. trachomatis* (say, >5 per cent incidence, and usually for those younger than 25 years), this verbal screen should be backed by DNA-based *Chlamydia* pre-screening. This can be as important for re-insertions as for initial IUC insertions.
> - Recent exposure history or evidence of a purulent discharge from the cervix indicates referral for more detailed investigation at a genitourinary

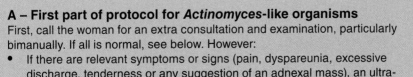

medicine (GUM) clinic. If *Chlamydia* is detected, the woman should be referred to a GUM service:
 — To be investigated for linked pathogens.
 — To have necessary treatment and contact tracing arranged, and
 — Usually to have the IUC insertion postponed.
• However, National Health Service (NHS) resources can be saved by not doing unnecessary testing for vaginal organisms. To quote the FSRH guidance, 'in asymptomatic women... there is no indication to test or treat other lower genital tract organisms'.
• In EC cases, screen – but either treat anyway before the result is available (e.g. with azithromycin 1 g stat) or (FSRH Guidance), if asymptomatic ensure the woman can be contacted and treated promptly in the event of a positive result.
• The cervix should be cleansed (primarily physically, removing mucus by swabbing) before any device is inserted, with minimum trauma, following the manufacturer's instructions.
• In addition to the routine 6-week follow-up visit, the woman should be given clear details of the relevant symptoms of PID and instructed as routine to telephone the practice nurse about 1 week after device insertion. This should identify any women with an early infection (during the crucial 20 post-insertion days of Figure 17).

The *Chlamydia* screen can be omitted if, for example, the woman is older than 35 years of age and the sexual history of 'mutual' monogamy is strong, particularly if her family is considered complete.

'Blind' prescription of an appropriate antibiotic can be appropriate in emergency cases, but the screening should still be done. Otherwise, contact tracing is impossible, and re-infection will simply occur later than the first 20 days (see Figure 17).

Actinomyces-like organisms

These organisms are sometimes reported in cervical smears – more commonly with long duration of use of either IUDs or IUSs.

If *Actinomyces*-like organisms (ALOs) are reported:

A – First part of protocol for *Actinomyces*-like organisms
First, call the woman for an extra consultation and examination, particularly bimanually. If all is normal, see below. However:
• If there are relevant symptoms or signs (pain, dyspareunia, excessive discharge, tenderness or any suggestion of an adnexal mass), an ultrasound scan should then be arranged to image any adnexal disorders, with a low threshold for gynaecological referral.

> - After preliminary discussion with the microbiologist, the device should be removed and sent for culture. Treatment will have to be vigorous, usually prolonged, if frank pelvic actinomycosis is actually confirmed – it is a potentially life-threatening and fertility-destroying condition, although very rare.

Much more usually, the ALO finding occurs in asymptomatic women who are free of physical signs – who stay that way. Over-reaction may cause more morbidity through pregnancy than through actinomycosis, given the latter's rarity.

In the second part of this protocol on detection of ALOs, when there are no positive clinical findings, in consultation with the woman the clinician may decide between either of the following approaches, B or C. Each approach has some supporting evidence. The FSRH Guidance favours C.

B – Second part of protocol for *Actinomyces*-like organisms
- Simple removal with or without reinsertion, and without antibiotics.
- Removal without reinsertion is advisable at or after the menopause, because of case reports of later IUC-associated frank actinomycosis (p. 162).
- Advise the woman, along with written reference material, about the relevant symptoms that are highly improbable but should make her seek urgent medical care and to tell the doctor that she recently had an IUD or IUS and monitoring for ALOs.
- Repeat a cervical smear after 3 months (it will nearly always be negative) with a re-check bimanual examination. Both smear taking and IUC follow-up then revert to normal.

C – Alternative protocol for *Actinomyces*-like organisms
- Leave the IUD or IUS alone after the initial thorough and fully reassuring examination.
- Advise the woman, and provide her as for protocol B with written material, about the relevant very rare symptoms that should make her seek a doctor urgently and to tell her or him that she is being followed up with an IUD or IUS and monitoring for ALOs.
- Arrange follow-up (which now is not done routinely for IUDs or IUSs), initially at 6 months, including a check for symptoms and bimanual examination as indicated, and then revert to normal 'open-house' follow-up (p. 133).

Is ectopic pregnancy caused by IUCs?

This is another IUC myth. The main cause of ectopic pregnancy is previous tubal infection, with damage of one or both tubes. The non-causative association with IUCs comes about because they are even more effective at preventing pregnancy in the uterus than in the tube.

Ectopic pregnancies are actually reduced in number, because very few sperm get through the copper-containing uterine fluids to reach an egg, so very few implantations can occur in any damaged tube. However, there are even fewer implantations in the uterus. Thus, in the observed ratio, the denominator of intrauterine pregnancies is reduced more than the numerator of ectopic pregnancies. So it is important to be aware, clinically, that ectopic pregnancies are definitely more likely to occur among the much-reduced number of IUC-related pregnancies – even though both types of pregnancy are actually reduced in frequency.

The estimated rate of ectopic pregnancy for sexually active Swedish women seeking pregnancy is 1.2 to 1.6 per 100 woman-years. The risk in Swedish users of either the T-Safe Cu 380A and its clones or the Mirena LNG-IUS is estimated as 0.02 per 100 woman-years, which is at least 60 times lower, thus confirming the foregoing argument.

Accordingly, UKMEC classifies a past history of ectopic pregnancy as WHO 1. Clinically, however, caution is necessary among current users of all IUCs (see Slogan 6), especially Jaydess, pending more data, which has a lower release of LNG: a higher ectopic pregnancy rate than the foregoing rate of 0.11 per 100 woman-years has been reported, and 50 per cent of the (very few) conceptions were ectopic.

> **IUC Slogan 6**
> Any user with pain and a late or unusually light period, or irregular bleeding with a positive pregnancy test result and no pain (yet), has an ectopic pregnancy until proved otherwise.

Moreover, because there are even better *anovulant* options (e.g. combined hormonal contraceptives [CHC], contraceptive implants (Nexplanon in the UK), or depot medroxyprogesterone acetate [DMPA]), in nulliparae generally a past history of ectopic pregnancy is WHO 3 (JG) for IUCs (see p. 129).

Pain and bleeding

As already stated in IUC Slogan 3 (p. 112) pain and bleeding in IUC users signify a dangerous condition – until proved otherwise (and then, indeed, in early days it may well prove to be reactive, especially in a nullipara, and respond well to analgesics). Besides excluding conditions such as infection or an ectopic pregnancy or miscarriage, consider malpositioning of the frame of an IUC, which can cause pain through uterine spasms. Beyond the first few post-insertion days, a well-located IUD rarely causes pain. The same is true for the IUSs which, moreover, over time often reduce pre-existing uterine pain particularly if associated with endometriosis.

Copper devices can be ideal, like reversible sterilization, for well-selected women with light menses. They need to know that:

- The duration of bleeding may increase, by a mean of 1 day.
- The measured volume of bleeding usually increases by about one third (yet this can be a hardly noticeable addition if the woman's normal periods are light, e.g. 20 ml increasing to 27 ml).

Bleeding problems usually settle with time. If they do not, it may be necessary to change the method of contraception – perhaps to an IUS (see later).

Drug treatments may reduce the loss, but are not very satisfactory in the long term. The most successful therapies are mefenamic acid 500 mg every 8 hours (which can simultaneously help pain as well and so is usually tried first) and tranexamic acid 1 to 1.4 g every 8 hours.

Duration of use

Studies regularly show reduced rates of IUC discontinuation with increasing duration of use – whether for expulsion, infection or pain and bleeding or indeed pregnancy. Coupled with the fact that most IUC complications are insertion related, it is good news that the banded devices T-Safe Cu 380A and clones may be used for 10 years or longer.

After the age of 40 years, the agreed policy, set by a 1990 statement in the *Lancet* by the Family Planning Association and the predecessor body of the FSRH, is as follows:

IUC Slogan 7

Any copper device (even a copper wire-only type) that has been fitted in a woman older than 40 years may be used for the rest of reproductive life (in practice, until no later than about 55 years; see p. 162).

It never needs replacement, even though it is not licensed for that long. For the duration of use of IUSs in various situations, see later.

LEVONORGESTREL-RELEASING INTRAUTERINE SYSTEMS (MIRENA®, LEVOSERT® AND JAYDESS®)

These LNG-IUSs are schematically depicted in Figure 18.

Method of action and effectiveness

LNG-intrauterine systems (Mirena and Levosert, also Jaydess)
The main points
- The standard LNG-IUS (in its two versions) contains 52 mg of LNG and initially releases about 20 µg/24 hours into the uterus from its polydimethylsiloxane reservoir, through a rate-limiting membrane.
- The daily release rate falls to a mean of 14 µg at 5 years – which is more than adequate. (Jaydess, the 13.5-mg LNG-IUS, is smaller and starts out with that 14-µg release rate, yet it is an effective contraceptive over 3 years).
- Its main contraceptive effects are local, through changes to the cervical mucus and utero-tubal fluid that impair sperm migration, backed by endometrial changes impeding implantation.
- Its cumulative failure rate to 7 years was very low, at 1.1 per 100 women in the large Sivin study – even less until its licensed 5 years in a European multicentre trial by Anderson *et al.*
- Its efficacy is not detectably impaired by enzyme-inducing drugs.
- The systemic blood levels of LNG are initially higher (explaining early hormonal side effects) but fall in the first 3 months to less than half of the

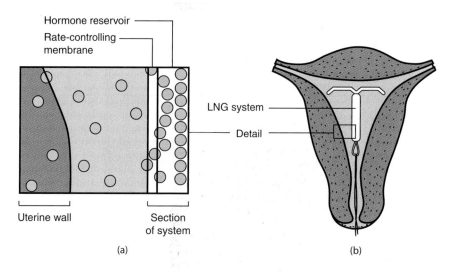

Hormone reservoir

Rate-controlling membrane

LNG system

Detail

Uterine wall

Section of system

(a)

(b)

Figure 18
(a) and (b) The intrauterine system (IUS). Applies to the 52-mg levonorgestrel-IUS and also (with slight differences shown in Table 10) to Jaydess®, which contains 13.5 mg.

mean levels in users of the LNG POP. A stable level is reached after about 3 months and can be described to users as 'roughly like taking three old-type POPs per week' – or about two a week with Jaydess (see later).

- The amount of LNG in the blood is still enough to give unwanted hormone-type side effects in some women; otherwise, irregular light bleeding is the main problem.
- Although ovarian function is altered in some women, especially in the first year, 85 per cent show the ultrasound changes of normal ovulation.
- Even if users become amenorrhoeic – as many do, primarily through a local end-organ effect – in those who do not ovulate (as well as the majority who do), sufficient estrogen is produced for bone health.
- Return of fertility after removal is rapid and appears to be complete.

Levosert®

Levosert is a 52-mg LNG-IUS that is new since the last edition. It is manufactured in a different facility from Mirena and feels palpably different to the touch, but has been shown to be fully bioequivalent. It differs mainly in the following ways:

- An inserter device with a 4.8-mm diameter tube. The (one-handed) Evo-inserter for Mirena has a 4.4-mm tube.
- Release of the IUS into the uterus is by the easy-to-learn two-handed technique, rather similar to that for the Nova T380.
- Not yet (2015) licensed for more than 3 years' use as a contraceptive, but this will increase: an ongoing efficacy study is to be continued to at least 7 years.
- Not yet (2015) licensed for endometrial protection in HRT.

Levosert is licensed for treating heavy menstrual bleeding as well as contraception, but for use during HRT it would be medico-legally safer (JG) to wait for full marketing authorisation.

Advantages and indications

The user of one of the 52-mg LNG-IUSs can expect the following advantages:

- The amount and, after the first few months (discussed later), duration of blood loss are reduced dramatically.
- Dysmenorrhoea is improved in most women.
- The 52-mg LNG-IUS is the contraceptive method of choice for most women with heavy menstrual bleeding, and it prevents or treats iron-deficiency anaemia. Indeed, it is still a first-line treatment, when contraception is not needed, for both heavy bleeding and menstrual pain (the latter even with normal blood loss).

- Endometriosis: Gynaecologists now recognize the LNG-IUS as often ideal for long-term maintenance therapy, after initial diagnosis and treatment.
- HRT: By providing progestogenic protection of the uterus during estrogen replacement by any chosen route, ideally non-oral so as to bypass the liver, the 52-mg LNG-IUS (as Mirena) offers unique advantages. Before final ovarian failure, the combination produces *contraceptive,* no-period and no premenstrual syndrome–associated HRT. For this increasingly popular indication, the Mirena IUS is *licensed* for 4 years; but there is now, since 2013, FSRH approval for replacement after 5 years (unlicensed; p. 165).
- Epilepsy: In a small series at the Margaret Pyke Centre in London, this was a very successful method in this condition, even in women on enzyme-inducer treatment.
- The 52-mg LNG-IUS is, in short, a highly convenient and 'forgettable' contraceptive – 'with added gynaecological value'.

The contraceptive advantages shown in the foregoing box are, of course, shared with the T-Safe Cu 380A, which is the current gold standard for copper IUDs. However, this is where the similarity ends. IUSs fundamentally 'rewrite the textbooks': they really share only the intrauterine location and certainly deserve a separate category (hence 'system' not 'device').

JAYDESS®

Launched in the United Kingdom in 2014, this is a smaller, 13.5-mg LNG-IUS, manufactured similarly to other IUSs but with a number of differences (Table 10). As compared with the 52-mg LNG-IUS (Mirena or Levosert) Jaydess has:
- A smaller diameter of its 'Evo-inserter', 3.8 mm versus Mirena 4.4 mm, so it is usually easier to fit through a tight cervix. Figure 19 neatly demonstrates this difference in the inserter tubes.
- Smaller dimensions: 28 versus 32 mm wide at the fundus, 30 versus 32 mm long. To assist imaging *in situ,* it also bears a small silver ring just under the arms of the T.
- Licensed for 3-year use, with initial release of 14-μg LNG/day versus 20 μg released by the 52-mg LNG-IUSs yet it has
- Comparably excellent efficacy and is
- Likely, although not yet proven, to cause fewer side effects from progestogen that enters the systemic circulation.
- Periods are observed to be likely to continue (although lighter than normal). A lower amenorrhoea rate than with 52-mg LNG-IUSs may (or may not) appeal to some women.

In summary, the 52-mg LNG-IUS is the more usual first choice, because of the following advantages over Jaydess (Table 10):
- Longer duration of use.
- Being licensed for use for heavy menstrual bleeding (HMB) and for endometrial protection during HRT.

However, Jaydess may be preferred by some. Indeed it could be an excellent alternative to Nexplanon® for some young women, including nulliparae, given that it may be easier to fit than the larger type of IUS and, in comparison with Nexplanon, the greater likelihood of an acceptable (regular, light) bleeding pattern. Jaydess is extremely unlikely to fail and is not believed to 'cause' ectopic pregnancies; but among the very few failures there is that 50 per cent risk of extrauterine conception (p. 119). So the user should have an advance briefing on the relevant symptoms (i.e. pain and irregular bleeding occurring without and even more so with a positive pregnancy test result).

Table 10

Two types of LNG-releasing intrauterine system. Images reproduced with permission of Bayer HealthCare.

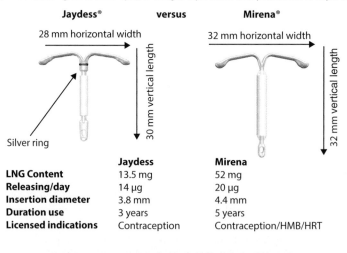

	Jaydess	Mirena
LNG Content	13.5 mg	52 mg
Releasing/day	14 µg	20 µg
Insertion diameter	3.8 mm	4.4 mm
Duration use	3 years	5 years
Licensed indications	Contraception	Contraception/HMB/HRT

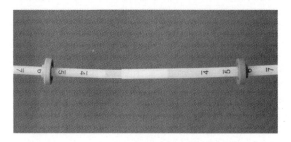

Figure 19

Demonstration of relative narrowness of the pink Evo-inserter tube of Jaydess (3.8 mm) in comparison with that for Mirena (4.4 mm). (Courtesy of Professor Anne MacGregor, and Colin Parker of Durbin PLC.)

What about infection or ectopic pregnancy risk and risk to future fertility?

Although IUCs do not themselves cause PID (see earlier), they fail to prevent it, and there is a suspicion that they sometimes worsen the attacks that occur. LNG-IUSs may reduce the frequency of clinical PID in long-term users, perhaps through the progestogenic effect on cervical mucus. Although the risk is certainly not eliminated, the available data make it possible to offer an IUS, or, indeed, a copper IUD – appropriately, after raising the issue of using condoms *as well* if and when there is STI risk – to many young women requesting a 'forgettable' contraceptive. Their future fertility is most unlikely to be adversely affected.

The data published for LNG-IUSs show (as with the banded copper IUDs) a massive reduction in ectopic pregnancy risk, which can be attributed to its great efficacy by the sperm-blocking mechanism that reduces the risk of pregnancy in any site. However, in the case of a past history of an ectopic pregnancy, an anovulant method would be even better than any IUS.

Problems and disadvantages of the IUSs

- Expulsion can occur as for any IUC.
- There is the usual circa 1–2 per 1000 risk of perforation, minimized by its 'withdrawal' as opposed to a 'plunger' technique of insertion.
- Pain suggests malpositioning: it is not expected, indeed pain is usually improved with an IUS. Check by ultrasound scan, ahead of insertion, whenever fibroids are suspected at the preliminary examination.
- A significant problem is the high incidence in the first post-insertion months of uterine bleeding, which, although small in quantity, may be very frequent or continuous and can cause considerable inconvenience. Forewarning about this is crucial.
- In later months, amenorrhoea is commonly reported – sometimes perceived as a problem, although it is really not so!
- Hormonal side effects are common in early months (see later).

Women can accept the early weeks of light bleeding, even if very frequent, as a worthwhile price to pay for all the other advantages of the method, provided they are well informed in advance of IUS fitting. They can be confident that perseverance will be rewarded because this early problem has such a good prognosis. If it does not settle or recurs later, the D-checklist (p. 59) has some relevance. Short-term use of a COC sometimes appears to help (no good evidence, but FSRH guidance is that this 'could be tried for up to 3 months'). Beyond 3 years of use, unexplainable bleeding that returns unacceptably may justify trying early replacement of any IUS.

Oligo-amenorrhoea can and should be interpreted to a woman as an advantage – thus gently debunking the myth that menstruation serves an excretory function – not an adverse side effect but a positive benefit of the method.

Women should also be forewarned that, although this method is mainly local in its action, it is not exclusively so. Therefore, there is a definite incidence of 'hormonal' side effects such as bloatedness, acne and depression. These do usually improve, often within 2 months, in parallel with the known decline in the higher initial LNG blood levels. Strangely, in comparative studies such 'hormonal' symptoms have not actually been proved to occur more often than in users of copper IUDs.

The frequency of developing functional ovarian cysts is also increased, although these cysts are usually asymptomatic. If pain results, the cysts should be investigated or monitored, but they usually resolve spontaneously.

Contraindications

Many of the contraindications of this method are shared with copper IUDs (see later). The additional few contraindications unique to IUSs are the result of the actions of its LNG hormone, some of which enters the systemic circulation, and they are discussed in the following box.

Unique contraindications (WHO group as stated) for the IUSs, among intrauterine methods
- Current breast cancer – This is WHO 4 according to UKMEC, with the IUS becoming usable on a WHO 3 basis after 5 years' remission, as with all the other progestogen-only methods. In my view:
  - Because IUSs give the lowest overall systemic hormone dose of such methods, and
  - Given the suggestive data that the 52-mg LNG-IUS may protect against tamoxifen-induced pre-cancer changes in the endometrium, in selected cases this WHO 3 status may be agreed considerably sooner, after consultation with the oncologist.
- Trophoblastic disease (any) – As for copper IUDs, this is WHO 4 while blood human chorionic gonadotropin (hCG) levels are high, but there is no problem (WHO 1) after full recovery (hCG undetectable).
- Current liver tumour or severe (decompensated) hepatocellular disease (WHO 3) or past CHC-related cholestasis (WHO 2).
- Gallbladder disease (WHO 2).
- Current severe active arterial or venous thrombotic disease, risk factors or predispositions (all WHO 2).

In addition, the IUS should not be used as a post-coital IUC (failures have been reported); acting hormonally, it appears not to act as rapidly as does the intrauterine copper ion.

Duration of use of the 52-mg LNG-IUS in the older woman

The Mirena 52-mg product is so far the only version licensed for 5 years
However, it should be noted:
- For contraception, effective use is evidence-based but unlicensed for up to 7 years. For a woman younger than 40 years, because of her greater fertility, replacement after the usual 5 years would be advisable. However, the older woman whose 52-mg LNG-IUS was fitted after the age of say 40 may continue to use it for 7 years, at her fully empowered request (but always on a 'named-patient' basis – p. 165). Furthermore, the FSRH guidance (2015) states that women who have the 52-mg LNG-IUS inserted at the age of 45 years or older for contraception can retain the device if amenorrhoeic until the menopause is confirmed, or contraception is no longer required (see Slogan 8).
- As part of HRT, the Summary of Product Characteristics (SPC) states that for safe endometrial protection the system should be replaced at 4 years, although the FSRH since 2013 has permitted use for 5 years (specifically for Mirena).
- However, if any LNG-IUS is not being and will not be used for either contraception or HRT, it could be left *in situ* for as long as it continues to work, in the control of heavy and/or painful uterine bleeding, and then removed after ovarian failure can be finally ensured. It should not normally be *in situ* beyond about age 55 years (actinomycosis risk; see p. 162), however.

IUS Slogan 8
Women who have the Mirena LNG-IUS inserted at the age of 45 years or more for *contraception* and are amenorrhoeic can retain their system until the menopause is confirmed or until contraception is no longer required – possibly up to about age 55, in fact (see p. 163).

Conclusions – the LNG intrauterine systems

This method fulfils many of the accepted criteria for an ideal contraceptive (see the box on p. 8). It approaches 100 per cent reversibility, effectiveness and even, after some delay, convenience. This is because, after the initial months of frequent uterine bleeding and spotting, the usual outcomes of either intermittent light menses or amenorrhoea are very acceptable to most women. Adverse side effects are few and, in general, are in the 'nuisance' category rather than hazardous.

However, this method does fail on some criteria: above all, it is not sufficiently protective against STIs, especially the sexually transmitted viruses, so wherever STI transmission risk applies, condoms must be used in addition. We also eagerly await an implantable version, based on the GyneFix concept.

CONTRAINDICATIONS TO INTRAUTERINE CONTRACEPTION – GENERALLY

Note that these apply primarily to copper IUDs but also to IUSs, except where stated. (The contraindications that are unique to the IUSs have already been listed.)

Absolute – but perhaps temporary – contraindications (WHO 4) to fitting all IUDs and IUSs
- Suspicion of pregnancy.
- Undiagnosed irregular genital tract bleeding, until the cause is known or treated as necessary.
- Significant current infection: post-septic abortion, current pelvic infection or STI, undiagnosed pelvic tenderness/deep dyspareunia or purulent cervical discharge.
- Significant immunosuppression.
- Malignant or benign trophoblastic disease, while hCG is abnormal (WHO 4 for IUDs and the IUSs, according to UKMEC). This is in case the uterine wall is invaded by tumour, thereby increasing the risk of a perforation. However, this becomes WHO 1 when hCG is undetectable.
- IUSs only: Breast cancer is UKMEC 4, and it becomes UKMEC 3 in remission (like the POP, p. 77, given that IUS-users do have some circulating progestogen). However, this may be an indication for a copper IUD.
- The woman's own ethical values forbid her to use a method with a possible post-fertilization mechanism (p. 108; see also p. 137).

Absolute permanent contraindications (WHO 4) to fitting IUDs and IUSs
- Markedly distorted uterine cavity, or cavity sounding to less than 5 cm depth (but this is only WHO 2 for GyneFix Viz).
- Known true allergy to a constituent of the product.
- Wilson's disease (copper IUDs only – this is precautionary advice, through absent data).
- Pulmonary hypertension, because of a significant risk of a fatal vasovagal reaction through cervical instrumentation.

Note that previous endocarditis and risk thereof are WHO 1, not now consid-ered contraindications, nor is any antibiotic cover routinely required for IUD or IUS insertions (see BNF Section 5.1).

Relative contraindications to intrauterine contraceptives – WHO 2 unless otherwise stated

This is a longish list, but in all cases meaning an IUD or especially an IUS is definitely usable, with some degree of caution.

1. Nulliparity and young age, especially less than 20 years. This combi-nation is WHO 2 because the actual insertion process is likely to be more difficult, and there are more serious implications should there be a severe infection (with no babies yet). However, WHO 2 does mean 'broadly usable'. Moreover, UKMEC classifies nulliparity after age 20 as entirely acceptable (WHO 1) for both copper IUDs (often inserted as EC; see Chapter 7) and the IUSs.

2. Lifestyle of self or partner(s) at high risk of STIs, or past history of pelvic infection. Combined with item 1, this may equate to WHO 3: if the method is even so chosen, there needs to be committed condom use.

3. Recent exposure to high risk of a STI (e.g. after rape). As EC, a copper IUD may be used (WHO 2) with full antibiotic cover (and after *Chlamydia* testing is done).

4. Known human immunodeficiency virus infection. While controlled by drug therapy, this is only WHO 2. An LNG-IUS is better still because of reduced blood loss (added condom use is routinely advised anyway).

5. Past history of ectopic pregnancy or other history suggesting high ecto-pic pregnancy risk in a nullipara is WHO 3, in my view (UKMEC is less cautious), but WHO 1 (as UKMEC) if there are living children. If used, banded copper IUDs or IUS are the best; but it is even better to use an anovulant method.

6. Suspected subfertility already. This is WHO 2 for any cause or WHO 3 if it relates to a tubal cause.

7. Post-partum: in UK insertion usually at 6 weeks, and WHOMEC warns it should not be earlier than 4 weeks during breastfeeding, when perfora-tion risk is increased up to 6-fold. So lactation is WHO 2 (proceed with caution) and not ideal for a teaching session!

8. Fibroids or congenital abnormality of the uterus with some but not marked distortion of the uterine cavity (see earlier). This is WHO 2 for framed IUDs or IUSs and WHO 1 for GyneFix Viz (only if inserted by an expert, because perforation risk is high when the cavity is distorted).

9. Severely scarred or distorted uterus (e.g. after myomectomy) (WHO 3).

10. After endometrial ablation or resection – there is a risk of the IUC's becoming stuck in the shrunken and scarred cavity. IUSs and GyneFix Viz are useable in selected cases.

11. Heavy periods, with or without anaemia before insertion for any reason, including anticoagulation. This is an indication for IUSs (WHO 1).

12. Dysmenorrhoea, any type. The 52-mg LNG-IUSs may well benefit all types and can indeed be used to treat pain in the absence of heaviness of bleeding.
13. Endometriosis. This may be benefited by the 52-mg LNG-IUS (WHO 1), to help local symptoms in addition to systemic treatment.
14. Previous perforation of the uterus. This is WHO 2, almost WHO 1, based on the small defect in the uterine fundus after a previous IUC perforation. Healing is so complete that it is usually difficult even to locate the site of the previous event.
15. Pelvic tuberculosis is WHO 3, or WHO 4 if future fertility is hoped for.

Notes
- If it is available and a copper IUD is desired, GyneFix Viz, being frameless, would often be preferable for items 8, 9 and 10.
- The IUSs may often be preferred or indicated, notably for the conditions listed in items 4 and 10 to 13.

COUNSELLING, INSERTION AND FOLLOW-UP

Timing of insertions – for all intrauterine contraceptives
- In the normal cycle, timing must be planned to avoid an already implanted pregnancy, but otherwise it is a myth that insertion is best during menses (higher expulsion rates are reported then, in fact, unsurprisingly, see below p. 131).
- With copper IUDs (because they are such efficient post-coital methods), insertion can be at any time up to 5 days after the calculated day of ovulation, or even:
- At any time in the cycle – if the provider is reasonably certain of the woman not having an implanted pregnancy in a conception cycle (see p. 158).
- For the IUSs, a more cautious timing policy is advised (see later).
- Post-partum insertions of IUDs or IUSs are usually at 6 weeks and are acceptable from 4 weeks (beware the reported increased risk of perforation [p. 129]). If the woman is not fully breastfeeding, conception risk should be discussed (pp. 158–61) – and with the IUSs, additional contraception is advised for 7 days.
- Following first-trimester abortion (but only after preliminary counselling and with full agreement by the woman), immediate insertion has been established – by systematic reviews and good studies – to be good practice (see Slogan 9). This means the immediate insertion being:
  - On the day of surgically induced abortion; or
  - After the second part of a medical abortion, if the uterus is clearly empty – this can be checked by on-the-spot ultrasound.

Additional points about insertion timing for any IUS

- In the normal cycle: Insertion for all IUSs should be no later than day 7 of the normal cycle, because it does not operate as an effective post-coital contraceptive and because, in addition, any fetus *could* be harmed by conception in the first cycle (given that there are known to be extremely high local LNG concentrations in the endometrium). Later insertion is acceptable, but only if there has been believable abstinence beforehand and with continued contraception (e.g. condoms) after IUS insertion, for 7 days.
- If a woman is on a CHC or POP/DSG POP or Nexplanon or DMPA, the IUSs can normally be inserted any time, with no added precautions. Preliminary 'bridging' with a quick-started COC or POP can be ideal (see below and p. 160).

Clinical implications

As for Nexplanon, insertions only in the foregoing tiny natural-cycle window are a logistic and conception risk nightmare! So a useful practical tip is to actively recommend at counselling, as normal routine, the use of an anovulant method (usually a COC or DSG POP), as a 'bridging' method (p. 160) from then until the LNG-IUS insertion. A pregnancy test at 3 weeks may be planned if this bridging method was quick-started later than Day 7. If not so, or if that test is negative, insertion can then be at mutual convenience, without any timing problems or conception anxiety.

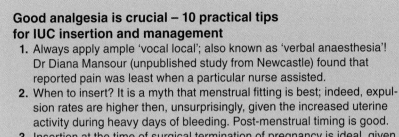

Good analgesia is crucial – 10 practical tips for IUC insertion and management

1. Always apply ample 'vocal local'; also known as 'verbal anaesthesia'! Dr Diana Mansour (unpublished study from Newcastle) found that reported pain was least when a particular nurse assisted.
2. When to insert? It is a myth that menstrual fitting is best; indeed, expulsion rates are higher then, unsurprisingly, given the increased uterine activity during heavy days of bleeding. Post-menstrual timing is good.
3. Insertion at the time of surgical termination of pregnancy is ideal, given the already present local or general anaesthesia. Misgivings about expulsion rates, infections and acceptability are without foundation. IUDs or IUSs can, and should, be offered to all women whose pregnancies end in the first or early second trimester. May this become the *norm*!

But only, of course, with full counselling and agreement well beforehand and definitely with easy opt-out.

4. Pre-medication should be routine approximately 40 to 60 minutes beforehand because there is evidence, for mefenamic acid 500 mg, that this helps to pre-empt the uterine cramping pain reported at 10 minutes after insertion. Naproxen 500 mg has also been shown to help this pain, but oddly not ibuprofen.

5. Local anaesthesia to the point of application of the tenaculum should be offered: 10 per cent lidocaine sprayed on the cervical surface has been reported (2015) to help, unlike surface gel application. This needs confirmation. Highly effective is a 1-ml dose of *warmed* lidocaine 1 per cent plain or e.g. prilocaine 4 per cent, injected *slowly* through the finest available needle, two minutes ahead. With attention to details, this procedure can be almost painless but it stops the unpredictable, sometimes (in about 10 per cent of women) very severe and continuing, sharp pain caused by the holding forceps. To offer this routinely (with opt-out) is arguably more important than using Instillagel® 2% lidocaine jelly, though the latter may help too – the evidence is mixed but suffices (JG's view), provided the provider:
   - Instils the gel slowly.
   - Stops stat when the woman reports any cramping.
   - *Waits* for its action: at least 3 minutes and in selected cases (e.g. past failed procedures) for more than 10 minutes.

6. Local anaesthesia injected paracervically at the level of the internal os is a very different procedure, needed only if the cervical canal needs dilation to Hegar 5 to 6.

7. Beware: Truly short cavities are rare. If the sound passes to less than 5 cm, it may have measured only the cervical canal.

8. Hard-to-display cervix? Try the left lateral position, which may also reduce speculum discomfort. This is a 'pseudo-lithotomy', if one adjusts insertion procedures through 90 degrees. Not ideal as a routine (loss of eye contact).

9. Insertion is considered 'complete' only after a satisfactory first follow-up, usually at 6 weeks. After that, however, routine annual check-ups are *not* required for any IUC, according to WHO (p. 133).

10. Above all, the IUC-provider – nurse or doctor – should:
    - Be well trained in using the different inserters (note that the Levosert inserter differs from the one-handed 'Evo-inserter'® for Mirena and Jaydess) and all ancillary equipment, including for 'lost threads'.
    - Stay competent by maintaining expertise.
    - Pay attention to detail.
    - Always be unhurried.

Counselling and follow-up

After considering the contraindications, there should be an unhurried discussion of all the main practical points about this method with the woman, focussing on infection risk and the importance of reporting pain as a symptom at any time – and of telephoning if it occurs in the early weeks after insertion.

The pre-insertion examination should be as already fully described, pp. 116–17, and she should always be given a user-friendly backup leaflet. She should be assured that during the use of the method, in the event of relevant symptoms or if she can no longer feel her threads, she will always receive prompt advice ('open house') and, as indicated, a pelvic examination.

The only important routine follow-up is the visit at about 6 weeks after insertion. This is to:
- Discuss with the woman any menstrual (or other) symptoms.
- Check for expulsion, including partial expulsion: The overall rate is about 4 to 5 per cent with all framed IUDs and the IUSs, mainly in the first 3 months.
- Exclude infection (i.e. no relevant symptoms, tenderness or mass).

IUC Slogan 10 – regarding follow-up
With IUDs and IUSs, until the first follow-up visit has happened, the insertion cannot be said to be complete. Thereafter, there should be no routine follow-ups, just 'open house' as noted in the next paragraph.

For 'open house' to work, all in the provider service must be in agreement that any IUC user will be sure to receive prompt help if she has symptoms, as given in the following box. Pain is the number one 'red flag' symptom in IUC users, with a serious cause (such as PID, ectopic pregnancy, malposition) until proved otherwise.

Reasons for an IUD or IUS user to seek urgent medical assistance
- Pelvic pain, low central or one-sided.
- Deep dyspareunia.
- Much increased or offensive discharge.
- Missed period.
- Significant menstrual abnormalities.
- Non-palpable threads (if could previously feel them) or overt expulsion.
- She or partner can feel the stem of partially expelled device.

Training for the actual insertion process

A book such as this is not the right medium for teaching insertion techniques. The FSRH training leading – now for nurses like doctors (p. 2) – to the Letter of Competence in IUC techniques is strongly recommended. This starts with e-learning on e-SRH (electronic sexual and reproductive health), followed by further self-directed theoretical training – and then practical training using a model uterus and culminating with at least seven competent insertions of copper IUDs and the IUSs. Full details are available at www.fsrh.org/pdfs/ IUT_TrainingRequirements.pdf

As we have already noted, it is worth getting all aspects of insertion training right, given the truth of IUC Slogan 1 (p. 109) – that insertion can be a factor in the causation of almost every category of IUC problems. The trainee's expertise must also be maintained thereafter through the FSRH's recommended *minimum* of one IUC insertion per month, on average.

Emergency contraception

There are two basic varieties of EC, initiated after unprotected sexual intercourse (UPSI):

- Copper ions, inserted as a copper IUD.
- Hormonal methods, taken by mouth.

Among the hormonal options, past methods included estrogens alone in very high dose and the combined oral emergency contraceptive (COEC) using LNG 500 μg and EE 100 μg repeated in 12 hours. Currently marketed hormonal EC methods in the United Kingdom are as follows:

- The levonorgestrel progestogen-only emergency contraceptive (LNG EC, Levonelle 1500® or Levonelle One Step®, also marketed as Upostelle®) in a stat dose of LNG 1500 μg.
- Ulipristal acetate (UPA, ellaOne®) in a dose of 30 mg.

Faculty of Sexual and Reproductive Healthcare (FSRH) Guidance on emergency contraception can be found at: www.fsrh.org/pdfs/CEUguidanceEmergencyContraception11.pdf.

COMBINED ORAL EMERGENCY CONTRACEPTION

Although COEC is no longer marketed in the United Kingdom as such, it is a useful though little-known fact that it can be constructed using the standard LNG 150 μg and EE 30 μg COC, which has at least 60 names and is marketed in almost every country on the planet. WHO advises four tablets of, for example, Microgynon 30 stat up to 72 hours after UPSI, repeated in 12 hours. It is rather sad to think of the number of women worldwide having unwanted conceptions because of ignorance in their society (and among providers) of this simple option, which they would have wanted to use.

COPPER INTRAUTERINE DEVICES

Mechanism of action

Insertion of a copper IUD – not the LNG-intrauterine system (IUS) (see p. 127) – before implantation is the most effective EC method available. Copper ions are immediately toxic to sperm and also prevent implantation. This means, after consultation with the woman, that insertion may proceed in good faith:

- Up to 5 days after the first sexual exposure (regardless of cycle length); and also
- Up to 5 days after the (earliest) calculated ovulation day.

This means working out, together with her:

- The soonest likely next menstrual start day, then
- Subtracting 14 days for the mean life of the corpus luteum, and
- Adding 5 days to allow for the shortest estimated interval from fertilization to implantation (Figure 20).

The judge's summing up in a 1991 court case (*Regina vs. Dhingra*) gives legal support to thus intervening up to 5 days post-ovulation or fertilization:

> *I further hold... that a pregnancy cannot come into existence until the fertilized ovum has become implanted in the womb, and that that stage is not reached until, at the earliest, the 20th day of a normal 28 day cycle...*

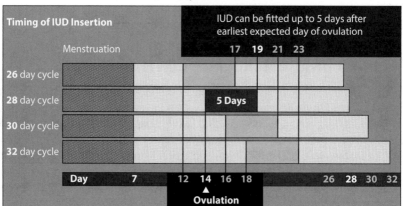

Where in the cycle can I fit an IUD?

NB: all to be in "utmost good faith", on both sides, including the coital and menstrual history

Figure 20
Use of copper as EC, relative to the calculated day of ovulation: regardless of number of previous episodes of UPSI.

Moreover, the UK Family Planning Association (FPA) convened a Judicial Review that also confirmed in 2002 the long-held position of most ethicists – namely, that a pregnancy begins at implantation, not when an egg is fertilized – and gave this concept *legal status* in the United Kingdom. It is also in my view (JG) *ethical*, since it is only after implantation that the chance of future life for any blastocyst exceeds *zero* (as argued on pp. 458–9 of *Contraception: Your Questions Answered,* 6th edition). However, some women still believe that any intervention after fertilization constitutes abortion, not contraception. That view must be respected in consultations (moreover, similar concerns can apply with respect to non-emergency – i.e. long-term use – of the IUD or IUS, p. 128).

Effectiveness of copper as emergency contraception

Women deserve to know that immediate insertion of a copper IUD is by far the most effective EC. **A 2012 systematic review reported a failure rate of approximately 1:1000,** even in cases of multiple exposure since the last menstrual period. Women who present almost always prefer an oral method, but in some circumstances they may need to be encouraged to consider this instead:

Indications for EC by copper IUD

IUD insertion may be preferable to oral EC:

- When maximum efficacy is the woman's priority – her choice. UKMEC says it should be *offered* to all – indeed, even to those presenting within 72 hours.
- Delay in presentation or multiple exposure. Insertion may be
  - Up to 5 days after the earliest UPSI at any time in the cycle, or
  - If there have been many UPSI acts, no later than 5 days after calculated ovulation (p. 136).
- In many women when the IUD is to be retained as their long-term method*. Always try to insert a banded IUD (e.g. the Mini TT 380 Slimline®) when long-term use is likely. However, if the internal os is tight, the Flexi-T 300® can be useful in the short term, or (better for the longer term) the UT 380 Short® (Figure 21 and see pp. 109–110).
- In the presence of contraindications to the hormonal method (unusual, but enzyme-inducer drugs are an example [WHO 3] – so consider an IUD, for e.g. a St John's wort user).
- If the woman is coincidentally suffering a vomiting attack when she presents, or unexpectedly and repeatedly vomits her dose of hormonal EC within 2 hours (for UPA, the Summary of Product Characteristics [SPC] says within 3 hours), in a case with particularly high pregnancy risk.

*Nulliparity does *not* rule out long-term use. Yet it may be appropriate, regardless of parity, to remove the IUD after the next menses – when the 'emergency' is over and the woman is established on a preferred new method, such as an implant (or switching to an IUS, if bleeding is a problem with the IUD).

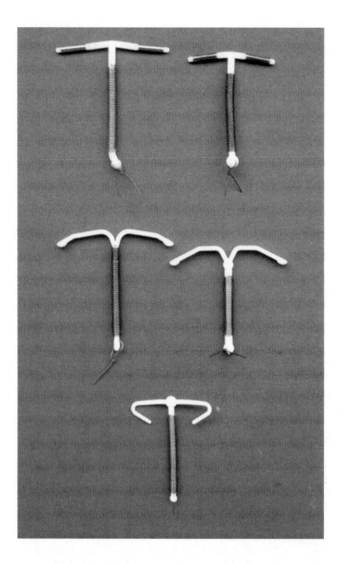

Figure 21

Recommended copper IUDs for use, in order of preference. (Courtesy of Professor Anne MacGregor, and Colin Parker of Durbin PLC.) Use lower order options if there is difficulty in fitting higher. Row 1: (first choice) T-Safe Cu 380A®, in any of its standard forms, or on right the TT Slimline Mini® which is smaller, but has similar insertion tube diameter (4.8 mm). Row 2: Nova T380®, Neo-safe T380® or UT 380 Standard® (all identical), or on the right the UT 380 Short®, recommended for a minimum uterine length of 5 cm. Inserter tube diameter for all these is 3.6 mm. Row 3: Cu-Safe T300® or Flexi-T 300® (identical). This has narrowest tube (3.5 mm) and a no-plunger insertion technique but is not preferred for long-term use because of a reported high expulsion rate, and it is also loaded with less copper than the above.

Contraindications to the IUD method and clinical implications

The IUD method has a number of recognized contraindications (pp. 128–30). and always risks short-term pain, bleeding or post-insertion infection, not to mention the inevitable 'hassle'. So this option needs to be provided well, despite the 'emergency'.

A good sexual history (see p. 7) should be taken from everyone presenting for EC, and UK studies suggest an above-average risk that such women are carrying *Chlamydia trachomatis.* If the sexual history is confirmatory and the woman agrees (after explaining, as one always should, the *relationship implications* should the test result be positive), she should be tested for gonorrhoea if that is locally prevalent, otherwise at least for this STI – maybe even if having hormonal EC. Warn also that recently acquired STIs may not be detectable until later retesting. If the result is not available before IUD insertion, there should be the following:

- Prophylactic antibiotic cover (e.g. with azithromycin 1 g stat) and
- Arrangements for contact tracing if STI test results later prove positive.

An *alternative*, preferred in FSRH Guidance, especially if the risk of infection is deemed low, is to treat only at early follow-up if the Chlamydia result comes back positive after the insertion. Insertion may be expected to be difficult sometimes, especially but not exclusively in nulliparae. Helpfully, the procedure rarely needs to be on the day of presentation. It can usually be arranged later after referral to a skilled colleague at a nearby service, given the ability to use IUDs later in the cycle, up to 5 days after ovulation (see earlier). Insertion could be on day 18, say, for a woman with a 27-day shortest cycle, presenting at a branch surgery on day 15 after high-risk UPSI repeatedly before that.

In such cases, the FSRH recommends giving hormonal EC on the day of presentation, as a holding manoeuvre.

HORMONAL EMERGENCY CONTRACEPTION

After sexual exposure, the earlier hormonal EC is given, the better – according to some but not all the studies. Yet **EC remains a better lay term than 'morning-after Pill'** because it leaves open two important facts – see box:

- Useful benefit can be obtained long after the 'morning after' – indeed the UPA hormonal method is licensed for use up to 5 days after sex (the *earliest* UPSI that cycle).
- There is a copper IUD alternative, which is not a 'Pill' at all.

Levonorgestrel emergency contraception

Dose: LNG 1500 µg stat within 72 hours of sexual exposure.

Mechanism of action

Given at or before ovulation, the LNG EC method

- Interferes with follicle development, either inhibiting it altogether or sometimes delaying ovulation – clinically, impress therefore on any user the continuing conception risk from unprotected sex after treatment.
- Possibly, of minor importance, makes the cervical mucus hostile to sperm.

However, given later in a cycle, after fertilization, LNG is now thought to have an almost negligible effect to prevent implantation. If there is thought to be the need for that mechanism, by far the most effective agent remains the copper ion.

Effectiveness and advantages

The apparent effectiveness of LNG EC with treatment up to 72 hours after a single sexual exposure is around 98% – but this represents prevention of only 70 to 75 per cent of the expected pregnancies because most women who present would not actually have conceived. Moreover, in the real world, multiple acts of UPSI without 'perfect' condom use both before and after the treatment can greatly increase the conception risk. This risk may be reducible by giving LNG EC more than once (in the same cycle) – which is endorsed by the FSRH although not yet licensed.

Emergency contraception with ulipristal acetate

Dose: UPA EC as ellaOne (HRA Pharma) 30 mg stat within 120 hours (5 days) of sexual exposure.

Mechanism of action

UPA is a synthetic selective progesterone receptor modulator with antagonist and partial agonist effects. Its primary mechanism of action is now known to be to delay ovulation until sperm from a sexual exposure (UPSI) are no longer viable. It does this even after the start of the LH surge.

Effectiveness

In a meta-analysis of two studies in which there was both abstinence and, crucially, no hormonal contraception until the next period, UPA EC prevented around twice as many pregnancies as LNG EC, and the best current estimate of actual conceptions prevented is approximately 85 per cent. It also has greater efficacy through until 120 hours after the earliest UPSI in that cycle. Hence, unlike LNG EC, it is fully licensed for use until then, 5 days after sex.

Without abstinence the failure rate of both EC methods has been shown to increase – 4-fold in the case of UPA EC: an argument at first glance for quick-starting (see pp. 159–60), that day, the woman's chosen long-term contraceptive. *However, since Sept 2015, if any progestogen-containing method follows after UPA EC, there is an **important new policy**, as now explained*:

More about hormonal ECs – which to use, why, and how?

1. Following UPA, a progestogen receptor *antagonist*, it was previously expected that all quick-started progestogen-containing contraceptives would have their effectiveness reduced. However two publications in 2015 [Cameron *et al.* Hum Reprod 2015;**30**:1566–1572; and Brache *et al.* Hum Repro 2015. doi:10.1093/humrep/dev241] found, first, that this effect on ovulation is NOT shown when desogestrel (DSG) is quick-started – which seemed good news. But there was more:

2. **UPA EC nearly always DELAYS rather than inhibiting ovulation.** Though LNG EC acts by delay less often, we should have been warning *all* EC-takers before now, *that 'after working fine today, there might be a fully fertile egg released during the next week'*.

3. Those data at 2 had seemed to reinforce the argument for quick-starts routinely after hormonal EC; that is, until Brache *et al.* in 2015 unexpectedly (to most of us) showed that, after UPA, the risk of a subsequent fertile ovulation in the next 5 days actually *increases highly significantly with next-day quick-starting of a DSG POP*. Sperm might easily survive in the genital tract till then.

4. The mechanism is thought to be that DSG reinitiates the ovarian progesterone receptor signalling that the antagonist UPA had blocked. There is concern (unconfirmed) that the same may well apply to all contraceptives containing a progestogen, DSG or other. Therefore, pending more data:

Clinical implications after UPA EC (only):

The FSRH advises (Sept 2015):

- *Do not start* ANY progestogen-containing method until 5 days later with (ideally) abstinence, or condoms till then,
- Continue the latter *for some days after the new FP method starts, as is usually advised* (the detail re number of days follows, here).
- Generally, when starting hormonal contraception later than the 5th day of a cycle, including quick-starting after LNG-only emergency contraception, FSRH Guidance advises condoms, or avoidance of sex, for 7 days for CHCs (9 days for Qlaira®), implants & injectables and 2 days for POPs. (But see Footnote on p. 82 re the latter advice).
- Therefore, following that 5-days of (solely) abstinence or barriers that is now advised after EC using UPA, extra precautions should continue for the same number of days as in last bullet after a progestogen-containing method is started.

So which hormonal EC should now be recommended?

There's been no change in the evidence that, *provided there is no quick-started hormonal method*, UPA EC is more effective (**x 2**) than LNG EC for UPSIs occurring before presentation. So, ***in high conception risk cases***:

- *UPA is clearly the 'stronger' EC IF* a woman accepts abstaining (ideally) for 5 days, and then continues so or uses condoms, well: either until her next period, or for some days fewer if she *'semi'-quick-starts* hormonal FP after 5 days.
- *Otherwise*, if (only if?) it is deemed unlikely she will fully comply with the instructions just given, and if the 'strongest' EC of all (*EC by Cu*) is unacceptable: 'apply clinical judgement' as the FSRH says about using LNG EC. After all, that method:
  − *does allow next-day quick-start of a new hormonal method and*
  − *after missed pills, allows immediate return to COC or POP.*

Other facts specific to UPA EC:

1. There is at least a 20% incidence of a week's delay in start of the next menses *even when the UPA EC 'works'* – no surprise given its mechanism, but women should be pre-warned about this....
2. It is not recommended for use *more than once* per cycle – an accepted though unlicensed practice with LNG EC – since unlike the latter there are no fully reassuring data, yet, re UPA not harming a fetus if the woman were to conceive.
3. UPA EC is also, of course, more expensive than LNG EC for the National Health Service, although it has been shown in two studies to be *cost effective*, primarily by preventing more conceptions.

Maintenance of efficacy

Enzyme-inducer drug treatment

If the woman is taking any one of these agents (listed on pp. 55–6, including St John's wort; also bosentan, p. 75), hormonal EC is WHO 3. As usual, WHO 3 means that it would be much better to use an alternative, ideally:

- Insertion of a copper IUD (which is completely unaffected by drugs).

If not acceptable, the choice is either

- LNG EC with the dose of LNG EC being doubled (i.e. two tablets totalling 3 mg stat [unlicensed use, p. 165 – but endorsed by the FSRH]) or:
- UPA EC with the dose doubled to 60 mg stat (JG). This is a biologically plausible but similarly unlicensed practice, and we need more clinical data. It is not yet in 2015 endorsed by the FSRH.

High body weight

Limited, not yet conclusive, data suggest that there may be reduced efficacy of hormonal EC with increased body weight, and that UPA EC may be more effective than LNG EC above about 75 kg. Pending more data, I therefore prefer UPA EC for patients weighing more than 75 kg (JG), while agreeing with the European Medicines Agency (EMA) and the FSRH that the potential benefits of any EC outweigh anything related to weight. (BMI is less relevant because the mechanism here probably relates to dilution of the hormonal EC in *total body water,* which is high in a heavy woman regardless of height.)

Contraindications to hormonal emergency contraceptives

WHO 4 conditions

There are vanishingly few WHO 4 conditions. Aside from current pregnancy when it would be redundant anyway, in my view (JG) these are as follows:

- Known severe hypersensitivity to a constituent (moderate or dubious allergy would be WHO 3).
- Known acute porphyria (WHO 3), although with greater reluctance if history of severe attack(s) induced by sex hormones. UKMEC says WHO 2, but my view (JG) is more cautious.
- If it emerges on discussion that the woman's own ethics preclude intervention post-coitally (or, more relevantly, post-fertilization – i.e. she disagrees with the UK legal view; see earlier).
- UPA is not currently recommended with severe hepatic impairment or in severe asthma treated by oral glucocorticoids.

Relative contraindications (WHO 3 or 2)

- Enzyme-inducer drug treatment; see earlier (WHO 3) – copper IUD preferred.
- Current breast cancer (WHO 2 because of uncertainty, but an adverse effect is unlikely with such short exposure).
- If a significant absorption problem is anticipated (WHO 2, or WHO 4 during ongoing acute vomiting).

Breastfeeding is not a contraindication, although the conception risk may often of course be so low (pp. 74, 156) that EC treatment would not be needed. If hormonal EC should be indicated, a risk to the infant from the small amount of UPA that enters the breast milk cannot yet be excluded. Given that the SPC for ellaOne advises no breastfeeding for 7 days, and that is likely to be an unacceptably long time to be expressing breast milk, pending more data it seems better to use LNG EC for these (infrequent) cases.

WHICH METHOD TO USE?

The FSRH Guidance (2012) states clearly that providers *'should inform women about the different methods with regard to efficacy,* adverse effects, interactions, medical eligibility and need for additional contraceptive precautions. The efficacy of UPA has been demonstrated up to 120 hours and *can be offered to all eligible women requesting EC during this time period'*.

If women are, as this proposes, routinely informed of the three EC methods, and they *decline a copper IUD,* is it not obvious that most will then request 'the morning after pill that works better'? The available data suggest that at all time intervals after UPSI UPA EC is more effective, so this guidance points to its use as the first choice in high conception-risk cases for all who will abstain, or use condoms well, till the next menses.

Any other indications? As we have seen, if it appears that EC will be given during the approximately 5 days between fertilization and implantation, the most effective course despite the perceived 'hassle' for all concerned is always copper IUD insertion. However, could UPA, with its anti-progestogen activity, be a new option here, so long as it is made very clear that it is definitely less effective than copper? Maybe, but this use based on the calculated ovulation day is controversial and unlicensed (p. 165). It should be recorded that the woman clearly understands there is some doubt about both of the following:

- UPA's effectiveness at this dosage for blocking implantation and:
- Its safety for a pregnancy if, inadvertently, it were given even later, after a conceptus had implanted.

SUMMARY: COUNSELLING AND MANAGEMENT OF EC CASES

First, evaluate the possibility of sexual abuse or rape. Then, in a context that preserves confidentiality – and feels that way to the client – using (crucially) a good leaflet, such as that of the FPA, as the basis for discussion, help the woman to make a fully informed and autonomous choice. This could be any of the three EC methods, or, for some women who present too late, taking no action at all (i.e. waiting 'with fingers crossed' for the next period).

Pharmacists may now (2015) sell either LNG or UPA EC *over the counter*. Best practice would be that they ensure adequacy of their own training; privacy when with the client; and good referral pathways to a clinical provider, as indicated: for a copper IUD – or, for the future, maybe an implant or IUS.

Clinical management

- Careful assessment of **menstrual/coital history** is essential. Probe for other exposures to risk earlier than the one presented with. Note: Ovulation is such a variable event and LNG EC and UPA EC are so safe that most women are best treated whenever they present – in the 'normal' cycle.
- **Assess contraindications** – The mode of action may itself pose the only contraindication or problem for some patients. It may sometimes be acceptable to a woman with these ethical concerns if it is clearly going to be given well before ovulation (moreover this will only be delayed if UPA EC used) and she can be sure it will be out of her body by implantation.
- Medical risks may be a concern, and they should be set out in the information leaflet that is given, especially:
  - **The failure rate** – Remind the woman that the figures relate to a single exposure. The failure rate is close to nil for the IUD.
  - **Teratogenicity** if there is a failure: this is believed to be negligible if EC hormones are given, as they should be, before implantation: because they cannot reach the unimplanted blastocyst in sufficient concentration to cause any effect. Follow-up of women who have kept their pregnancies has so far not shown any increased risk of major abnormalities above the background rate of 2 per cent.
  - **Ectopic pregnancy** – If this follows after either hormonal or copper EC, as it may, the EC was not causative. It can occur only in a tube with pre-existing damage and would have happened anyway, with or without this (pre-implantation) EC treatment. However, a clear past history of ectopic pregnancy or pelvic infection remains a reason for specific forewarning with any EC method, and all women should be warned to report back urgently if they get *pain.* Also, providers must 'think ectopic' whenever EC by hormones or by copper may have failed, or there is an unusual bleeding pattern after treatment.
- **Side effects:**
  - With LNG EC in the WHO 2002 trial, nausea occurred in 15 per cent and vomiting in 1.4 per cent of users. If the contraceptive dose is vomited within 3 hours, before resorting to an IUD the woman may be given a further tablet with an anti-emetic: the best seems to be domperidone (Motilium®) 10 mg.
  - With UPA, in the RCT comparing with LNG EC (Glasier *et al. Lancet* 2010;375:555–562), all reported symptoms were similar (e.g. vomiting, 1.5 per cent), with no statistical differences.
- **Future contraception**, both in the current cycle (in case the LNG EC or UPA EC merely postpone ovulation) and in the long term, should be discussed. The IUD option covers both aspects (for a suitable long-term user). Inform the woman that using EC every month is not advised: during a year of monthly hormonal EC there is a higher risk of failure than by regular use of almost any approved method. If the COC or other medical method is chosen, it has in the past been started as soon as the woman

The foregoing description highlights the importance of a good rapport to obtain an honest and accurate coital or menstrual history, so as to proceed in good faith and also promote more effective contraception in future.

FOLLOW-UP

Women receiving LNG EC or UPA EC who do not quick-start a new method rarely need to be seen again routinely, but should be instructed to obtain advice

- If they experience pain, or
- If their expected period is more than 7 days late, or lighter than usual.

IUD acceptors return usually in 4 to 6 weeks for a routine check-up; or sometimes for device removal, now they are established on what for them is a more appropriate long-term method.

SPECIAL INDICATIONS FOR (HORMONAL) EC

These indications apply to coital exposure when the following have occurred:

- **Omission of anything more than two COC tablets after the Pill-free interval (PFI),** or of more than two Pills in the first seven of the following packet – *using LNG EC* (pp. 141–2), since the woman will normally return directly to a hormonal method. As explained on p. 45, *after* the first Pill-taking week, since seven tablets have been taken to render the ovaries quiescent, Pill-omissions almost never indicate emergency treatment. Moreover, towards the end of a packet (Pill-days 15–21), simple omission of the next PFI without EC will always suffice – no matter how many Pills have been missed, up to seven anyway!

- **Delay in taking a POP tablet for more than 3 hours**, outside of lactation, implying loss of the mucus effect, followed by sexual exposure before mucus-based contraception could have been restored. The POP is restarted immediately after the LNG EC, the preferred method, and extra precautions advised. As discussed in the Footnote on p. 82, the FSRH currently says this need only be for 2 days, but I now prefer to advise 7 days, as in the SPCs.
- **If the user of any POP is breastfeeding**, EC usually by LNG (p. 143) would be indicated only if either the breastfeeding or the POP taking were unusually inadequate (p. 74)!
- **Removal or expulsion of an IUD** before the time of implantation, if and only if another IUD cannot be inserted, for some reason.
- **Further exposure in the same natural cycle** (e.g. from failure of barrier contraception more than 2 days after a dose of hormonal EC has been taken). Additional courses of LNG EC are supported by the FSRH, 'if clinically indicated', given reasonable precautions to avoid treating after implantation (yet repeated use thereafter will not induce an abortion). This use is, again, outside the terms of the licence (see p. 165). Repeated use of UPA in this way is not currently advised.
- **Overdue injections of DMPA with continuing sexual intercourse**. See pp. 87–88 regarding when this indication may be appropriate, generally using LNG EC or sometimes a copper IUD.
- **Advanced provision of hormonal EC**: The FSRH supports this in selected cases, to increase early use when required (e.g. when travelling abroad, to cover the possibility of UPSI through condom non-use or rupture or even rape).

In all circumstances of use of EC, the women should be aware (as stated in the FPA leaflet) that
- The method might fail.
- It is not an abortifacient.
- It is given too soon to be able to harm a baby.

Other reversible methods*

BARRIER METHODS

Barrier methods are not yet out of fashion! In spite of well-known disadvantages, they all (above all, condoms) can provide useful protection against STIs. All users of this type of method should be informed about emergency contraception (EC), in case of lack of use or failure in use. Guidance documents are available from the FSRH at www.fsrh.org.

Vegetable- and oil-based lubricants, and the bases for many prescribable vaginal products, can seriously damage and lead to rupture of rubber: baby oil destroys up to 95 per cent of a condom's strength within 15 minutes. Beware of *ad hoc* use of, or contamination by, substances from the kitchen or bathroom cupboard! The following box lists some common vaginal preparations that should be regarded as unsafe to use with rubber condoms and diaphragms, but it is not a complete list. Water-based products such as KY Jelly®, and also glycerine and silicone lubricants, do not harm latex, but all oils and creams should be regarded as suspect.

Preparations known or presumed to be unsafe to use with rubber condoms or diaphragms

Arachis (peanut) oil	Gyno-Daktarin® (Janssen-Cilag)
Baby oil	Nizoral® (Janssen-Cilag)
Canesten® (Bayer and generic)	Ortho-Gynest® (Janssen-Cilag)
Cyclogest® (Actavis)	Ovestin® (MSD)
Dalacin® cream (Pharmacia)	Petroleum jelly
Gyno-Pevaryl® (Janssen-Cilag)	Sultrin® (Janssen-Cilag)
E45®, Dermol® and similar emollients (see British National Formulary [BNF])	Vaseline® (Elida Fabergé)
	Witepsol-based preparations

---

* See note re male and female sterilization at end of this chapter.

Condoms

Condoms are the only proven barrier to transmission of HIV – yet, at the time of writing, it still remains impossible in the United Kingdom for most couples to obtain this life-saver free of charge from every general practitioner (GP). Condoms are second in usage to the Pill among those younger than 30 years and second to sterilization in those older than 30.

One GP reported a failure rate as low as 0.4 per 100 woman-years, but a rate of 2 to 15 is more representative. Failure, often unrecognized at the time, can almost always be attributed to incorrect use – mainly through escape of a small amount of semen either before or after the main ejaculation. Conceptions – particularly among the young or those who have become a bit casual after years of using a simple method such as COC – can sometimes be 'iatrogenic' simply because of lack of explanation of the basics by a clinician or pharmacist.

Some users are entirely satisfied with the condom, whereas others use it as a temporary or backup method. For many who have become accustomed to alternatives not related to intercourse, it is completely unacceptable. Some older men, or those with sexual anxiety, complain that its use may result in loss of erection. I (JG) consider that this sometimes gives entirely sufficient grounds to prescribe a phosphodiesterase type-5 inhibitor (see BNF). For women who dislike the smell or messiness of semen, the condom solves their problem.

True rubber allergy can also occur (rarely), and it can easily be solved by switching to a modern plastic condom.

Plastic condoms

These condoms have become both cheaper and less intrusive for coital sensations. They have no latex smell and are intrinsically non-allergenic. Oils do not affect plastic condoms made from polyurethane or the synthetic resin AT10 used in Pasante Unique®. But polyisoprene, used in Durex Latex Free® and Mates Skyn® condoms, is a synthetic latex. With these condoms, oils are still best avoided. Although oils are less damaging to synthetic latex than to ordinary latex, in experiments oils make the condoms stretch, so theoretically more likely to slip off.

Femidom®

Femidom is a female condom comprising a polyurethane sac with an outer rim at the introitus and a loose inner ring, whose retaining action is similar to that of the rim of the diaphragm (Figure 22). It thus forms a well-lubricated secondary vagina. Available over the counter, along with a well-illustrated leaflet, it is completely resistant to damage by any chemicals with which it may come in contact. During use, the penetrative phase of intercourse can feel more normal to the male partner and can also start before his erection is

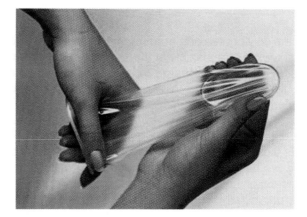

Figure 22
The female condom (Femidom®). (Courtesy of Chartex International PLC.)

complete. However, couples should be forewarned to avoid having the penis wrongly positioned between the Femidom sac and the vaginal wall.

Reports about the acceptability of Femidon are mixed, and a sense of humour certainly helps. There is evidence of a group of women (and their partners) who use it regularly, sometimes alternating with the male equivalent ('his' night, then 'her' night). Others might also choose it, if it were more often mentioned by providers as even being an option. As the first female-controlled method with high potential for preventing HIV transmission, it must be welcomed.

The cap or diaphragm

Although now considered 'old hat' and rarely used, many couples, once initiated, are pleasantly surprised at the simplicity of these vaginal barriers, although they are often acceptable only when sexual activity takes place in a relatively regular pattern in a long-term relationship. These devices may be inserted well ahead of coitus and so used without spoiling spontaneity. There is very little reduction in sexual sensitivity because the clitoris and introitus are not affected.

Spermicide is recommended because no mechanical barrier is complete, although we still lack definitive research on this point.

Possible toxic effects of nonoxinol-9 to the vaginal wall have become a real concern (see later). However, the vagina is believed to be able to recover between applications when nonoxinol-9 is used in the manner, and at the kind of average coital frequency, of typical diaphragm users. The lactic acid-based products mentioned below are alternatives with lower potential for irritation.

The acceptability of the diaphragm itself depends on how it is offered. Its first-year failure rate, now estimated as high as 6 per 100 careful and consistent users, rising to 16 per 100 typical users (see Table 1, p. 9), makes it very unsuitable for most young women who would not accept pregnancy. However, it suits others who are 'spacers' of their family. And it is capable of excellent protection in women older than 35 years (3 per 100 woman-years, as the Oxford/Family Planning Association (FPA) study reported in the early 1980s), provided it is as well taught and correctly and consistently used as it was by those couples. The Caya® contoured diaphragm is new to United Kingdom since the last edition and comes in one size to fit most women, but it has a reported first-year failure rate with consistent use of 13.7 per cent. Full details are at www.fsrh.org/pdfs/NewProductReviewCaya.pdf.

Since 2007, FemCap® has been the only cervical cap on the UK market. Intended for provision through mainstream family planning clinics (supplier: Durbin), it is a useful alternative to the diaphragm, although in a randomized controlled trial its 6-month failure rate was significantly higher, 13.5 per cent compared with 7.9 per cent for diaphragm users. It is a plastic cervical cap with a brim filling the fornices (displayed on right in Figure 1, p. 3) and comes in three sizes, thus substituting for previously available cervical caps. It must be used with a spermicide but is reusable, with replacement recommended about every 2 years. More details at: www.fsrh.org/pdfs/FemCapFinalGP.pdf.

When there is great difficulty in inserting anything into the vagina – be it tampon, pessaries or a cap – the method is obviously not suitable. This problem may be connected with a psychosexual difficulty that may first manifest during the teaching of the method, but simple lack of anatomical knowledge is often involved. Some training in these methods helps most women, though Caya is sold with no advice to involve a healthcare provider.

Follow-up
The fitting of diaphragms should be rechecked routinely post partum, or if there is more than a 3-kg gain or loss in weight.

If either partner returns complaining that he or she can feel any kind of cap during coitus, the fitting must be checked. It could be too large or too small; or with the diaphragm the retro-pubic ledge may be insufficient to prevent the front from slipping down the anterior vagina; or, most seriously, the item may be being placed regularly in the anterior fornix. The arcing spring diaphragm is then particularly useful.

Chronic cystitis may be exacerbated by pressure from a diaphragm's anterior rim. A smaller size may help. The condition was shown to occur less frequently with FemCap in the comparative pre-marketing trials.

For nurses or doctors who wish to offer this choice, there is no substitute for one-to-one training, both in the process of fitting a diaphragm or FemCap and in teaching a woman how to use it correctly.

With these products, the single most important thing the woman must learn is the vital regular secondary check, after placing it, that she has covered her cervix correctly. A small group of usually older couples, who must accept the far higher risk of contraceptive failure than with any LARC, say, can and do use these methods successfully. High motivation is essential. Once again, a good sense of humour helps.

Spermicides

Sadly, many useful products such as Delfen® foam and the Today sponge products have been removed from the UK market. Spermicide brands available (2015) are shown in Figure 1 (p. 3) on the right (tubes with applicator). Brands include Gygel® (with nonoxinol-9) and Caya Gel® and Contragel®. The latter products are sperm-immobilisers rather than destroyers, yet the intrinsic effectiveness of lactic acid has not been shown to differ from nonoxinol-9. These are options for women of reduced fertility when a male or female condom is unacceptable (see the following box).

Although invaluable as adjuncts to caps and diaphragms, when used alone spermicides often fail because they do not reliably deal with a whole ejaculate. Yet spermicides can be used successfully by women if – and only if – their natural fertility is reduced (see the following box).

A vaginal spermicide introduced through its applicator may be a satisfactory choice (although 100 per cent effectiveness is never on offer):
- During full lactation (LAM, p. 156) as an alternative adjunct to the POP.
- For women over 50 years of age for 1 year after periods cease (when contraception is still advised), whether or not they use HRT.
- For women aged over 45 with secondary amenorrhoea (contraception being required for 2 years before menopausal infertility can be diagnosed).
- During continuing secondary amenorrhoea at a younger age, unless a COC is being used anyway to treat hypo-estrogenism.
- As an adjunct to other contraception. Spermicides may rarely be suggested as a supplement in couples who are keen to continue using withdrawal as their main method: they need to know that the withdrawal must still continue. This is just extra 'to deal with any leakage').

Many substances are well absorbed from the vagina, but there is no proof of systemic harm, congenital malformations or spontaneous abortions through the use of current spermicides, chiefly nonoxinol-9 or its close relatives.

Occasionally, nonoxinol-9 causes irritation or allergic reactions, which are much less frequent with the lactic acid-based products above. More seriously, when used by Nairobi prostitutes four times a day for 14 days, nonoxinol-9 released from pessaries caused erythema and colposcopic evidence of minor damage to the vaginal skin.

Coupled with the doubts about its effectiveness against intracellular virus, it clearly should not be promoted as an anti-HIV virucide (see the systematic review by Wilkinson D, *et al. Lancet Infect Dis* 2002;2:613–617). However, pending better alternatives, for the time being it remains good practice to continue to recommend nonoxinol-9 for normal contraceptive use (less frequently than four times a day!), but not with condoms.

> **Final comment on spermicides**
> Worldwide, there remains an unmet need for an effective user-friendly female-controlled vaginal microbicide, which may or may not also be a spermicide. Progress is slow in this urgent and previously very neglected area of research.

FERTILITY AWARENESS AND METHODS FOR NATURAL REGULATION OF FERTILITY

At one time, these methods were generally despised and adopted only by those with strong religious views. Modern multiple index versions (based primarily on carefully charting changes to cervical mucus, the cervix itself by auto-palpation and body temperature, with support from the so-called secondary indicators such as ovulation pain) are popular among those who prefer to use a more 'natural' method. There is no space here to do justice to this approach, but there are extremely useful websites: www.fertilityuk.org. and also www.fsrh.org/pdfs/CEUGuidanceFertilityAwarenessMethods.pdf.

Those who wish to use these methods deserve careful explanation and ideally one-to-one teaching, particularly about charting the cyclical changes and the possible added use of other minor clinical indicators of fertility. Useful instruction leaflets, further advice and details of natural family planning (NFP) teachers available in different localities, can be obtained from www.fertilityuk.org (and also from the FPA website: www.fpa.org.uk). Additionally, these sources give advice about fertility awareness to assist conception.

With 'perfect use', the multiple index methods are capable of being acceptably effective. However, in the words of Professor Trussell of Princeton, they still remain 'very unforgiving of imperfect use'. Moreover, imperfect use is unfortunately common in the real world. To be effective, many days of abstinence are inevitable, and the highest possible cooperation from both parties is required but often lacking – especially from the male partner, whose motivation may well be suspect. (In one study, the failure rate was noted to be higher when the man rather than his partner was the one in charge of interpreting the temperature charts!) To be fair to the methods, failures also commonly result from poor use of other contraceptives, such as the condom, by those who do not wish to abstain during 'unsafe' days.

Standard days method (marketed as CycleBeads®)

This method is marketed as CycleBeads (see Figure 1, top right). For women with regular cycles, this is the calendar method reinvented for simplicity, using a ring of beads with different colours, one bead for each day of the cycle. There is a tight rubber band that should be moved daily over the beads, starting with the red one for day 1 of the period. Days 8 to 19 inclusive are white and signify 'no unprotected sex' (they are usefully luminous in the dark!). Proponents claim that although no adjustments are made for the given cycle being shorter or longer than 28 days this is balanced by easier compliance.

This has WHO 'modern method' status because there is evidence that, with consistent abstinence except on brown-bead days, the failure rate can be as low as 5 per cent after 1 year of use. However, careful identification of likely good users is absolutely crucial because in trials the failure rate was up to three times higher with 'typical' use. If users' ethics permit, condoms may be used on white-bead days, but although this increases acceptability, it also increases the failure rate. The method should moreover not be used by women who record cycles outside the range of 26 to 32 days.

See also the box on greater efficacy with these methods on p. 155.

Persona® (Unipath Ltd; Figure 23) is a combination of minilaboratory and microcomputer. It displays the 'safe' (green) and 'unsafe' (red) days of a woman's cycle, based on measurements of the first significant rise in her levels of urinary estrone-3-glucuronide and luteinizing hormone. With a reduced number of 'unsafe' days (8 to 10 for most women) being signalled per cycle, this contraceptive option is found by many couples to make things easier – but it does not apparently lead to greater effectiveness than careful charting of the indices with good compliance. The data on the failure rate are reported as 6 per 100 woman-years in the first year even with 'perfect use' – and Trussell (personal communication, 2003) still considers this to be an underestimate.

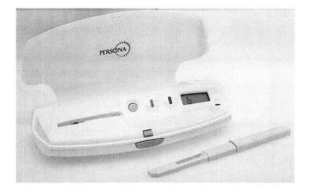

Figure 23
Persona®. (Courtesy of Unipath Ltd.)

Even on that slightly uncertain basis, couples should be informed that this is the same as a 1 in 17 risk of conceiving in the first year – on the high side, but perhaps good enough for 'spacers of their family.'

For greater efficacy with all these methods, couples should be advised to do the following:
- Use condoms on the pre-ovulatory days (the first sequence of brown-bead days with CycleBeads, or the first 'green-light days' if using Persona) – this being what I prefer to call the 'amber' phase (always less 'safe' because of the capriciousness of sperm survival in a woman).
- Abstain completely on all peri-ovulatory days (white-bead days, or 'red days' with Persona).
- Have unprotected intercourse only in the post-ovulatory phase (i.e. not until the fourth day after 'peak mucus', or in the second brown-bead or second green-light phases). Multiple indices are always safer, hence it would also add efficacy to have unprotected sex only after observing the *last* of the signals being used.

If Persona or another NFP method is to be commenced after any pregnancy or any hormone treatment – even just one course of hormonal EC – reliability demands that another method such as condoms or abstinence must first be used until there have been two normal cycles of an acceptable length (23 to 35 days).

Lactation within the specific guidelines of the lactational amenorrhoea method (LAM) as shown in Figure 24 constitutes a quintessentially 'natural method' – through to 6 months post-partum. It can be made even more effective by adding a POP p. 74).

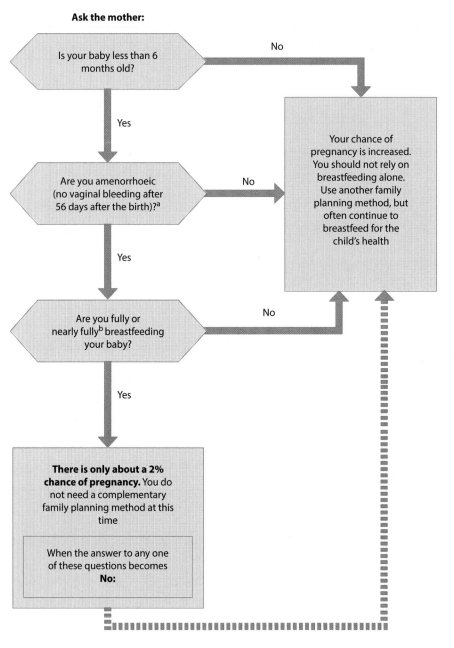

Ask the mother:

Is your baby less than 6 months old?

No

Yes

Are you amenorrhoeic (no vaginal bleeding after 56 days after the birth)?[a]

No

Yes

Are you fully or nearly fully[b] breastfeeding your baby?

No

Yes

Your chance of pregnancy is increased. You should not rely on breastfeeding alone. Use another family planning method, but often continue to breastfeed for the child's health

There is only about a 2% chance of pregnancy. You do not need a complementary family planning method at this time

When the answer to any one of these questions becomes **No:**

[a]Spotting that occurs during the first 56 days is not considered to be menstruation.
[b]Nearly full breastfeeding means that the baby obtains 100% of its nutrition from the mother alone, some water is allowed but certainly no solid food.

Figure 24
Algorithm for the lactational amenorrhoea method (LAM).

MALE AND FEMALE STERILIZATION

Sterilization, especially male sterilization, which is about five times as effective, after sperm counts have been done, as female sterilization with clips, is a useful option for selected couples, but not being reversible it is not within the remit of this chapter. For more, see my book with Professor Anne MacGregor: *Contraception: Your Questions Answered* (2013, Elsevier). Yet we argue there the case for generally preferring a long-acting reversible contraceptive (often an IUS or IUD) instead, for that finite, often quite short, time between ending childbearing and Nature's sterilization method, the menopause. Relevantly, when either one of the couple is sterilized, unacceptable menstrual symptoms often return on discontinuation of the combined hormonal contraceptive or other hormonal method. This is how *'vasectomy can cause menorrhagia!'* Certainly, whenever sterilization is mooted, one should never omit to ask all women about their periods as they were before hormonal contraception, maybe many years before. If they were troublesome (sometimes in the history they were actually put on the Pill decades earlier to control their menses!), a levonorgestrel IUS may well be altogether better than sterilization, whether for the male or female.

For much more on both male and female sterilization, including Essure®, the transcervical method using tubal inserts placed hysteroscopically and requiring, usually, only local anaesthesia or sedation, see the information from the FSRH at www.fsrh.org/pdfs/MaleFemaleSterilisation.pdf.

In comparison with laparoscopic sterilization using clips, clients should know that:

- Success with Essure always needs confirmation by hystero-salpingogram after 3 months and
- There is a 10-fold increase in failure or complications requiring re-operation (absolute risk about 2%). Mao *et al*. BMJ 2015;373:h5162.

HOW CAN A PROVIDER BE REASONABLY SURE THAT A WOMAN IS NOT PREGNANT, OR JUST ABOUT TO BE PREGNANT, IN A CONCEPTION CYCLE?

The World Health Organization on page 372 of its excellent publication *Family Planning: A Global Handbook for Providers* (2011 update – see p. 168 for full reference), advises that 'the provider can be reasonably certain that the woman is not pregnant if she has no symptoms or signs of pregnancy and if one or more of the following criteria apply':

1. 'Believable' abstinence since the normal last menstrual period (LMP).
2. Within 7 days of the normal LMP (less if short cycles; use judgement).
3. Within 4 weeks post-partum (not lactating).
4. Within 6 months post-partum with full breastfeeding and amenorrhoea (lactational amenorrhoea method [LAM]).
5. Within 7 days of abortion or miscarriage.
6. 'Believable' consistent use of a reliable contraceptive (may include condoms).
   To these 6, JG adds a seventh criterion:
7. In an oligo-amenorrhoeic woman older than 50 years (clinical judgement required).

Good clinical judgement is vital with respect to assessing the accuracy of the given history, including the following:

- The absence of symptoms of pregnancy.
- The believability of reported abstinence, especially regarding point 6 in the foregoing list: the reliability of reported correct condom use is notoriously difficult to assess.

In the United Kingdom, these criteria can be reinforced by a urine pregnancy test with a sensitivity of at least 25 IU/litre, but only if more than 3 weeks have elapsed since the last UPSI. Such tests are not helpful if there could not possibly yet be an implanted blastocyst present – including, for example, at the time of most requests for EC with a normal LMP.

SOME APPLICATIONS OF THE FOREGOING CRITERIA

Quick-starting and bridging

Background

Traditionally, initiation of hormonal and intrauterine methods of contraception has been delayed until the next menstrual period, mainly to avoid inadvertent use during pregnancy. However, that risk if a medical method is started at the time the woman is first seen can be minimized by a careful sexual and menstrual history. Moreover, according to the WHO:

- The risks to a fetus (i.e. of birth defects) from CHC or POP exposure are now known to be negligible or absent.
- Yet, it should be recorded that she has been *warned to stop promptly if she conceives* (i.e. before organogenesis – which occurs after the time of the first missed period). Ceasing then makes fetal damage even less likely.
- Record also the advice: '100 per cent follow-up to confirm not pregnant' – usually by text, e-mail or telephone, to the Practice Nurse. Should there be the slightest doubt, a pregnancy test is performed at least 3 weeks after the last UPSI – and at retail outlets such as 'Poundland' this now costs under £1.
- The main thing is that starting the new method only at the next period risks an avoidable conception *after* she was seen. The WHO, after reviewing all relevant data, concluded that this tradition *potentially causes more morbidity through conceptions than quick-starting or bridging, as defined in items 1 and 2 in the list in the next section.*
- Less important but useful, the woman is *probably* more likely actually to start and continue the new method now, when seen, than at the next period, especially if quick-starting after hormonal EC.

Clinical points

The box on p. 160 is adapted by JG from the FSRH Guidance, available at www.fsrh.org/pdfs/CEUGuidanceQuickStartingContraception.pdf. NB. With respect to quick-starting after ellaOne (ulipristal acetate) emergency contraception, note the important change in advice for women since 2015 (discussed at pp. 141–2).

1. If a health professional is *'reasonably sure'* (see the box on p. 158) that a woman is not pregnant from recent UPSI or on the way to conceiving (i.e. an unimplanted blastocyst), 'medical' methods of contraception can be started immediately (i.e. **'quick-started'**), unless the woman prefers to wait until her next period. Such practice for drugs or devices is usually unlicensed (p. 165). For ALL hormonal methods, the woman must also receive the usual advice when starting late in a cycle, about abstinence or condom use (see pp. 45, 56–7, 63, 69, 70, 79, 82, 86, 101 & 131).

2. **Bridging** is the same, except that – often because her preferred contraceptive is not available at first contact – the woman quick-starts usually with a pill (POP or COC), but plans with her FP provider, from the start, for this to be short term and to switch later, usually to a LARC.

3. *Avoid* generally this way of commencing:
   - **Anti-androgens:** drospirenone (as in Yasmin® and Daylette®, pp. 61–2), dienogest in Qlaira® and nomegestrol acetate in Zoely® (pp. 63–4) are about one third the potency of cyproterone acetate (in co-cyprindiol®, p. 62). With all these progestogens, there is uncertainty about the possibility of feminizing of a fetus, if it were to be male and continue to term.
   - **Levonorgestrel intrauterine systems** (LNG-IUSs) (Mirena®/Jaydess®), because if there should be conception, despite application of those WHO criteria (see p. 158), the peri-fetal concentration of LNG would be locally extremely high. (These levels of LNG are not dangerous to the uterus, but there is no certainty that they would not potentially cause some risk to the fetus.)
   - *Caution* also with DMPA, by either of now two routes (pp. 83–5): because, unlike all other methods, once injected, DMPA cannot be discontinued. Yet available data do suggest that a pregnancy is unlikely to be harmed by DMPA, so the decision to quick-start may be acceptable, on a case-by-case basis.
   - In all these cases, *initial bridging by POP or regular-type COC until conception can be confidently excluded is preferable* – even ideal (since it then allows any-day fitting of IUSs at mutual convenience).

4. The copper-bearing IUD may always be started immediately if the criteria for its use as EC are met (see pp. 136–7) with the great advantage that it also 'bridges' to the next period with, in suitable cases, long-term use to follow. This can be good practice for many nulliparous women.

5. Quick-starting, usually next day, after hormonal EC is often good practice; but this should only now occur using the LNG EC method. If ellaOne (UPA EC) is first used, no progestogen-containing method should follow until 5 days later with (ideally) abstinence, or condoms, till then. This is explained on pp. 141–2.

6. Quick-starting/bridging with usually a COC or the POP (e.g. DSG POP) can be part of a most useful *'ploy'* – see box on p. 161 – whenever there is amenorrhoea with recent or ongoing UPSI:
   - After a very overdue DMPA injection, defined by the FSRH as more than 2 weeks late (pp. 87–8); or
   - During post-partum amenorrhoea when the post-partum criteria of WHO in the box earlier in this chapter are *not* fulfilled.

If pregnancy is diagnosed and the woman wants the pregnancy to go to term, in all cases any quick-started or bridging method should be ceased, ideally just after the first missed period (i.e. before organogenesis).

What is the [JG] bridging 'ploy'?

Negative pregnancy test result at the time or not, the woman agrees to take (note: *really well*) the chosen anovulant pill with usual extra precautions initially as instructed – and then to have a follow-up pregnancy test after 3 weeks from the last UPSI. A negative result establishes no conception (whether implanted or unimplanted, at that time or indeed when she had first been seen), and she may then move to using any LARC.

CONTRACEPTION FOR THE OLDER WOMAN

Maximum age for COC use

Smokers of 15 or more cigarettes a day (or other women with a single strong arterial risk factor) should always discontinue the CHC at age 35 years (i.e. WHO category 3 becoming WHO 4) because excess mortality is detectable above that age, mainly from acute myocardial infarction. UKMEC allows women who stop smoking to continue on CHCs (WHO 3 falling to WHO 2 if they have abstained for more than 1 year). However, I say, in most cases, why, given the safer (LARC) alternatives now available?

If however she is a healthy, totally risk factor–free woman (e.g. migraine-free, normotensive, non-smoker) and is provided with modern Pills and careful monitoring, she may consider that the gynaecological and other benefits of CHCs outweigh for her the small, although increasing, cardio-vascular and breast cancer risks (pp. 17–19 and pp. 28–31, respectively) of the method until well beyond age 40 years. Although even for these women there could be better contraceptive choices, an appropriate CHC (prefer-ably the natural estrogen–containing Zoely or Qlaira, normally displacing now the usual 20-µg EE products) may be used in the late 40s (WHO 3). For healthy women with diminishing ovarian function but who need contra-ception as well, this may be preferable to standard hormone-replacement therapy (HRT) along with having to use some other contraceptive.

Beyond 50 to 51 years of age, the mean age of the menopause, the age-related increased CHC risks are usually unacceptable for all, given that fertility is now so low that simple, virtually risk-free contraceptives will suffice.

Most forms of HRT are not contraceptive but may be indicated, along with any simple contraceptive, in symptomatic women when estrogen is no longer being supplied by the COC. Of course, the Mirena IUS-plus-HRT combination is a winner here because it safely supplies contraceptive HRT with endometrial protection and, usually, also highly acceptable oligo-amenorrhoea (see the following box).

**The actual and expected advantages of HRT by Mirena LNG-IUS20®
plus natural estrogen** (p. 123) are:
- Contraceptive HRT for up to 5 years (p. 126).
- No-period, usually no-bleeding HRT – before proof of ovarian failure.
- Thus no heavy or painful loss HRT or PMS or other menstrual symptoms.
- Minimal systemic progestogen HRT.
- Still giving the expected quality-of-life benefits of HRT.

Diagnosing loss of fertility at the menopause

Although hormonal methods do mask the menopause, it is not always necessary to know the precise time of final ovarian failure. Unfortunately, for diagnosis of complete loss of ovarian function, FSH levels are essentially useless on their own. So one of the options in the following boxes should be used.

Plan A
**Contraception may cease: after waiting for the 'officially approved'
year of amenorrhoea after age 50, after having stopped all hormones**
This is the obvious plan for the following:
- Copper IUDs*.
- Condoms or a vaginal barrier method.
- Spermicide gel by applicator (which, unlike in younger women, may well suffice [p. 152] after age 50 when combined with oligo-amenorrhoea, although no one can be promised 100 per cent effectiveness).

*IUDs (and IUSs) should be removed 1 year after the final bleeding episode: if these devices are left *in situ* for many years post-menopausally, there have been case reports of severe actinomycosis and of pyometrium.

But what to do if the woman is using one of the hormonal methods or HRT, which mask the menopause?
- If on DMPA or an EE-containing COC (or other CHC): age 50 to 51 is the time to stop these. They are needlessly strong, contraceptively, and the known risks increase with age. Zoely and Qlaira are possible exceptions

to this (see p. 64), usable if requested on a WHO 2 basis (JG – but unlicensed, see p. 165) through to age 55 (see later).

- The POP, or an implant, or an LNG-IUS with or without HRT: As contraceptives these add negligible medical risks that increase with age, although the IUS, like IUDs, should be removed when not needed (actinomycosis risk, see the earlier box).
- Therefore, one of these (commonly a POP, not necessarily with DSG) may be continued until the latest age of potential fertility has been reached: then the woman simply stops the menses-masking contraception (no tests!). This is Plan B, as follows:

When is the latest fertile age?
A good estimate is age 55 years. The FSRH (see www.fsrh.org/pdfs/ContraceptionOver40July10.pdf) states that 'natural loss of fertility can be assumed by then for most women' – and this is confirmed if there is then continuing amenorrhoea. However a small minority, of the order of 4 per cent (a figure based on work in the 1960s so it may now be a few percentage points more, given greater average health these days) may menstruate beyond 55 years. Fertility of such cycles would obviously be very low, since the bleeding would very likely occur without a preceding fertile ovulation, but it cannot be guaranteed to be nil.

Plan B can therefore be:
Continue with a safe but period-masking contraceptive regimen (duration of any HRT is a separate issue), **until age 55, the latest age of potential fertility:** *then just stop that contraception.* No FSH or other tests. Most women will never see another period.

Yet it is essential to suggest use by all women of a simple method for *at least* 8 weeks. Gygel spermicide by applicator should suffice because of minimal residual fertility at this age (p. 152). Those few women who have bleeding episodes in that time (or, as they must be instructed, report any bleeding episodes later) are advised to:
- Continue with Gygel spermicide by applicator or use of condoms and report back when their periods *finally* seem to have ceased. Or, they may:
- Go back on a POP, which has virtually no known risks up to almost any age.

Plan B appears to be acceptably secure, but no absolute guarantees can be given: the *Guinness Book of World Records* has reported some exceptionally rare cases of motherhood without medical intervention beyond age 55 years.

Note that *neither* Plan A nor Plan B proposes using FSH for any guidance about final ovarian failure.

A third option, Plan C (JG), is intended for continuing users of a hormonal method who have started their sixth decade and want to learn sooner than by Plan B whether they may – or contrariwise *should not* – stop contraception (see the following box).

Plan C
Plan C is to ascertain whether four things apply to the patient:
1. She has *passed age 51,* **and**
2. She develops *vasomotor symptoms* after a trial of discontinuation of all hormones for *at least* 8 weeks, while abstaining or using condoms (spermicide not yet having been established as sufficient for that individual's fertility), **and**
3. *FSH levels measured twice are both high* (>30 IU/litre) – six weeks apart in the presence of flushes (unlike in other contexts, if items 1 and 2 are both true, FSH levels *are* usefully confirmatory), **and**
4. The *amenorrhoea continues* up to and beyond this trial period.

Along with due warnings (as usual) of lack of 100 per cent certainty, this protocol allows some women to cease all contraception earlier than by following Plan A or B. They should understand that even now to follow the one year rule of Plan A would be 'safer still'.

However, *if* any of these four do *not* apply, including that she has a later bleeding episode, the woman should continue or immediately restart appropriate contraception. This may have to be for some years because it implies that her own loss of fertility is coming later (than the mean age of about 51 years). If she is keen to avoid coitally-related methods, a good choice may commonly be a POP and the use of Plan B through to age 55 (or an earlier re-try of Plan C). However if methods that do not mask true amenorrhoea are acceptable, she could of course continue them until her periods cease completely (for 1 year, according to Plan A).

For COC users and POP users, there are a couple of useful clues that discontinuation of their method is worth a try, but then using for confirmation the Plan C or B protocol as given earlier:

- If COC users start getting 'hot flushes' at the end of their Pill-free interval – especially if a high FSH result is obtained then.
- If continuing users of POPs develop vasomotor symptoms with amenorrhoea (see p. 88).

Finally, should there be any doubt about the normality of any bleeding during these plans, investigate it – as always – as post-menopausal bleeding (PMB), to exclude malignancy.

Appendix

USE OF LICENSED PRODUCTS IN AN UNLICENSED WAY ('OFF-LABEL USE')

Often, licensing procedures have not yet caught up with what is widely considered the best evidence-based practice. Such use is legitimate and may indeed be necessary for optimal contraceptive care, whether by doctors *or* nurse practitioners in sexual and reproductive health (SRH), provided certain criteria are observed. These are well established. A useful acronym is **'EG-RY-PU-RB', as follows:**

1. **E**vidence **G**ood (best if endorsed by a Guidance document from a recognized authority such as the Faculty of Sexual and Reproductive Healthcare or National Institute for Health and Clinical Excellence).
2. **R**esponsibility **Y**ours – Pharmaceutical companies have no interest if the practice is not in their Marketing Authorization/Summary of Product Characteristics.
3. **P**atient **U**nderstands that this course of action, although evidence-based, is not yet licensed, and her informed verbal consent is best recorded. Yet: '...where prescribing unlicensed medicines is supported by authoritative clinical guidance, it may be sufficient to describe in general terms why the medicine is not licensed for the proposed use'. This explanation should usually be backed by written details (e.g. 'take two pills not one', 'run packets together, no breaks').
4. **R**ecords **B**rilliant – plus the treatment plan communicated to relevant colleagues, as appropriate.

Note: Attention to all the foregoing details is important – should harm be alleged, the manufacturer will claim no involvement.
The above is derived from General Medical Council: *Good practice in prescribing and managing medicines and devices*, paras 67–74. See: www.gmc-uk.org/guidance/ethical_guidance/14327.asp.

SOME 'BELIEVABLE' WEBSITES IN REPRODUCTIVE HEALTH

www.margaretpyke.org
Margaret Pyke Centre: Local services for London, contraceptive research and superb training courses on offer.

www.who.int/reproductive-health
World Health Organization: WHO's latest eligibility criteria and new practice recommendations.

www.ippf.org
International Planned Parenthood Federation: On-line Directory of Hormonal Contraceptives, the brand names used worldwide. Also many useful publications.

www.rcog.org.uk
Royal College of Obstetricians and Gynaecologists: Evidence-based College Guidelines on gynaecological topics interfacing with this text (e.g. infertility and menorrhagia).

www.fsrh.org:
Faculty of Sexual and Reproductive Healthcare of the Royal College of Obstetricians and Gynaecologists: Includes open access to Faculty Guidance pdfs on all methods plus numerous related topics (e.g. quick-starting, peri-menopausal contraception, drug interactions); access to the Journal; UKMEC tables; and more.

www.nice.org.uk
National Institute for Health and Care Excellence: Particularly useful in this context for its LARC Guideline.

www.fpa.org.uk
Family Planning Association: Patient information and essential leaflets.

www.brook.org.uk
Brook: Similar to the FPA website but for persons younger than 25; plus a secure on-line enquiry service. Helpline: 0800 0185023.

www.bashh.org
British Association for Sexual Health and HIV: National guidelines for the management of all STIs and a listing of GUM Clinics in the United Kingdom.

www.gmc-uk.org/guidance/ethical_guidance
General Medical Council: *'0-18 years guidance for all doctors'* – ethical guidance on all that relates to this age group.

www.likeitis.org.uk, www.sexunzipped.co.uk, www.nhs.uk/conditions/contraception-guide/pages/what-is-contraception.aspx, www.scarleteen.com
All these are user-friendly, accurate, and empowering for young people accessing sexual and reproductive health services and information.

www.familylives.org.uk (formerly parentline plus)
Family Lives: 'Top tips for parents'. How to help teens and pre-teens avoid many kinds of grief.

www.ecotimecapsule.com
John Guillebaud's 'Apology to the Future' project and his TED lecture 'Sex and the Planet', a catchy song "The Promise" – and more.

www.populationmatters.org
John Guillebaud's *Youthquake* document and much else of crucial importance to the planet's future.

For mail order supplies (e.g. for condoms; FemCap®; Caya® diaphragm; latest intrauterine devices and systems):
Durbin 020 8869 6590 (www.durbin.co.uk): Williams Medical Supplies 01685 844739 (www.wms.co.uk/fpsales)

www.condomoutlet.co.uk: mail order for most brands including important options in oil-resistant non-latex condoms.

FURTHER READING

Briggs P, Kovacs G, Guillebaud J (eds). *Contraception: a Casebook from Menarche to Menopause.* Cambridge: Cambridge University Press, 2013.

Cooper E, Guillebaud J. *Sexuality and Disability.* London: Radcliffe Publishing, 1999.

Guillebaud J, MacGregor A. *The Pill and Other Methods: The Facts.* 7th ed. Oxford: Oxford University Press, 2009.

Guillebaud J, MacGregor A. *Contraception: Your Questions Answered.* 6th ed. Edinburgh: Elsevier (Churchill-Livingstone), 2012.

McVeigh E, Homburg R, Guillebaud J. *Oxford Handbook of Reproductive Medicine and Family Planning.* 2nd ed. Oxford: Oxford University Press, 2012.

WHO. ***Family Planning: A Global Handbook for Providers (2011 update)*** Baltimore and Geneva: CCP and WHO, 2011. This is also freely downloadable from www.fphandbook.org/sites/default/files/hb_english_2012.pdf.

Other relevant titles, as well as DVDs and useful leaflets concerning individual methods and related topics, can be downloaded or obtained by mail order from the UK Family Planning Association (FPA) and the International Planned Parenthood Federation (IPPF). See their websites in the earlier list.

GLOSSARY

13.5-mg LNG-IUS	generic abbreviation used here and by the FSRH for the Jaydess IUS, containing 13.5 mg of LNG
52-mg LNG-IUS	generic abbreviation for the Mirena and Levosert IUSs
ALO	Actinomyces-like organisms
AMI	acute myocardial infarction
BBD	benign breast disease
BMD	bone mineral density
BMI	body mass index
BNF	British National Formulary
BP	blood pressure
BTB	breakthrough bleeding
CHC	combined hormonal contraception/ive
CIN	cervical intraepithelial neoplasia
COC	combined oral contraception/ive
COEC	combined oral emergency contraceptive
CPA	cyproterone acetate
CSM	Committee on the Safety of Medicines (UK)
CVS	cardiovascular system
DFFP	Diploma of the Faculty of Family Planning and Reproductive Healthcare, now the DFSRH

DFSRH	Diploma of the Faculty of Sexual and Reproductive Healthcare
DM	diabetes mellitus
DMPA	depot medroxyprogesterone acetate
DNA	deoxyribonucleic acid
DoH	Department of Health (now termed DH)
DSG	desogestrel
DSP	drospirenone
E_2	estradiol
EC	emergency contraception
EE	ethinylestradiol
EMA	European Medicines Agency
EVA	ethylene vinyl acetate
FAQ	frequently asked question
FDA	Food and Drug Administration
FH	family history
FP	family planning (method))
FPA	family planning association
FSH	follicle-stimulating hormone
FSRH	Faculty of Sexual and Reproductive Healthcare, formerly Faculty of Family Planning and Reproductive Healthcare
GP	general practitioner
GSD	gestodene
GUM	genitourinary medicine
hCG	human chorionic gonadotrophin
HDL	high-density lipoprotein
HIV	human immunodeficiency virus
HMB	heavy menstrual bleeding
HPV	human papillomavirus
HRT	hormone replacement therapy
HS	haemorrhagic stroke
HUS	haemolytic uraemic syndrome
IPPF	International Planned Parenthood Federation
IS	ischaemic stroke
IUC	intrauterine contraceptive/ion
IUD	intrauterine device
IUS	intrauterine system (generic term)
LAM	lactational amenorrhoea method
LARC	long-acting reversible contraceptive (method)
LH	luteinizing hormone
LMP	last menstrual period
LNG	levonorgestrel
LNG-IUS	levonorgestrel-releasing intrauterine system (used here to refer to either of two 52-mg LNG products)

LOC	Letter of Competence
MFFP	Membership of the Faculty of Family Planning and Reproductive Healthcare
MFSRH	Member(-ship) of the Faculty of Sexual and Reproductive Healthcare
MHRA	Medicines and Healthcare Products Regulatory Agency
MPC	Margaret Pyke Centre
NDFSRH	Nurse Diploma of the Faculty of Sexual and Reproductive Healthcare
NET	norethisterone (termed norethindrone in the United States)
NETA	norethisterone acetate
NFP	natural family planning
NGM	norgestimate
NHS	National Health Service
NICE	National Institute for Health and Care Excellence
OR	odds ratio
PCOS	polycystic ovarian syndrome
PFI	pill-free interval
PID	pelvic inflammatory disease
PIL	patient information leaflet
PMB	post-menopausal bleeding
PMDD	premenstrual dysphoric disorder (US term for severe PMS)
PMS	premenstrual syndrome
POP	progestogen-only pill
RCGP	Royal College of General Practitioners
RCT	randomized controlled trial
SDI	sub-dermal implant
SHGB	sex-hormone–binding globulin
SLE	systemic lupus erythematosus
SPC	Summary of Product Characteristics (= Data Sheet)
SRE	sex and relationships education
SRH	Sexual and Reproductive Health
STI	sexually transmitted infection
SVT	superficial vein thrombosis
TIA	transient ischaemic attack
TTP	thrombotic thrombocytopenic purpura
UKMEC	UK adaptation by the Faculty of SRH, of WHO's Medical Eligibility Criteria for contraceptive use
UPA	ulipristal acetate
URL	Uniform Resource Locator - on the internet
UPSI	unprotected sexual intercourse
VTE	venous thromboembolism

VVs	varicose veins
WHO	World Health Organization
WHOMEC	WHO Medical Eligibility Criteria for contraceptive use
WHOSPR	WHO's Selected Practice Recommendations for contraceptive use
WTB	withdrawal bleeding

Index

Note: Page numbers ending in "f" refer to figures. Page numbers ending in "t" refer to tables.

W

Weight gain, 1, 59–60, 89, 94, 104; *see also* Body weight
WHO, *see* World Health Organization
WHOMEC, *see* World Health Organization Medical Eligibility Criteria
Withdrawal bleeding (WTB), 13, 43–52, 55, 63, 70, 90, 103; *see also* Bleeding
World Health Organization Medical Eligibility Criteria (WHOMEC), 10–11
World Health Organization (WHO), 4, 10–11, 15
WTB, *see* Withdrawal bleeding

Y

Yasmin, 16, 24, 33–35, 53, 60–62

Young people
  contraception methods for, 4–7
  emergency contraception for, 4–7
  sex and relationships education for, 4–7
Young women
  breast cancer and, 17
  choices for, 4–7
  diaphragms and, 151
  hormonal contraception and, 68–69
  LNG-IUSs and, 124–125
  sex and relationships education for, 4–7
  taking 'breaks,' 67–68

Z

Zoely, 3f, 63–64, 160